THE GAUNTLET OF CAREGIVING

A GUIDE TO SURVIVE THE HEALTHCARE, GOVERNMENT, LEGAL AND COMPLEX ROLES OF FAMILIAL CAREGIVING

S.A. SAMS

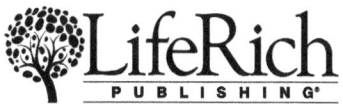

LifeRich Publishing is a registered trademark of The Reader's Digest Association, Inc.

LifeRich Publishing books may be ordered through booksellers or by contacting:

LifeRich Publishing
1663 Liberty Drive
Bloomington, IN 47403
www.liferichpublishing.com
844-686-9607

ISBN: 978-1-4897-5065-5 (sc)
ISBN: 978-1-4897-5063-1 (e)

Library of Congress Control Number: 2024910954

Print information available on the last page.

LifeRich Publishing rev. date: 10/30/2024

CONTENTS

DEDICATION

As humans that walk this earth for a short period of time, we are blessed to connect with others who inspire us, challenge us, help lift us, and teach us. I dedicate this book to all of those who have done these things for me in my lifetime. We often never know how we touch others in our life journey. Thank you all. I pray you know who you are.

To my Mother who chose life for me and set examples for me to follow and grow.

To my Mother-in-Law who has inspired me and is one of the most giving caregivers I know.

To my Husband who has challenged me in so many good ways, supported and loved me along each path.

To my Son who is a blessing, an inspiration, and has taught me so much.

DISCLOSURE/DISCLAIMER: The author nor anyone associated with this writing or publication is or claims to be an attorney or is providing legal advice. The information within this writing is strictly an opinion of definitions based on experiences and/or experiences from others shared with the author. No part represents specific people or situations and should not be construed as sharing personal information or outside the laws of any State or Central Government. Any commonalities felt are strictly because we are all touched by the human experience of caregiving at some point in our lives. The Gauntlet of Caregiving has no affiliation with any organizations mentioned and is not responsible for the content of their information materials or websites.

INTRODUCTION

"We are like books. Most people only see our cover,
the minority read only the introductions,
many people believe the critics.
Few will know our content."
– Émile Zola

As I arrived at the hospital which was in a town approximately twenty-five miles north of where I lived, it occurred to me that I was facing a situation that had not been a consideration in my life, for some odd reason. My Mom was in the hospital for an unknown issue. About an hour before a frantic friend of hers had called me saying, "The medics are here and they want to use the paddles on your Mom, is that ok?"

HUH? My brain said, "YES" I almost screamed into the phone. It was only later the reason for this call was revealed. A little red sticker on the refrigerator that said "DNR."

I had no idea until this moment that my Mother's life could so simply be ended.

4 Hospitals stays in 3 Weeks, in 3 towns,
… A Gauntlet

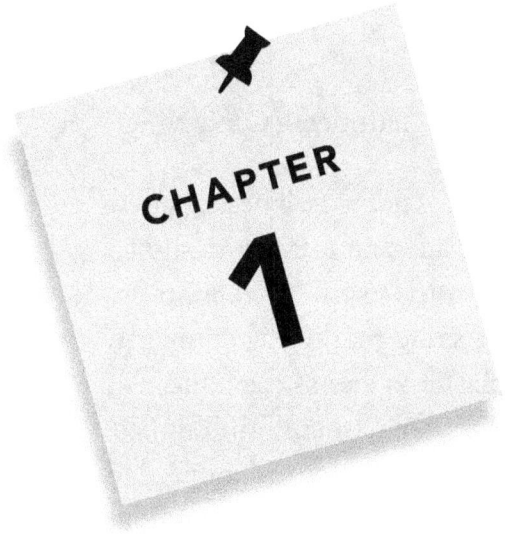

CHAPTER

1

Welcome to the Gauntlet of Caregiving

So glad you are here!

Yes, I became a Caregiver for a loved one, my Mother, in lightning speed. From experience and stories shared with me over the last fifteen years or so, I began to realize it can happen at any moment to anyone. One minute you are on vacation and a call comes in to describe an unbelievable situation when a loved one has been stricken with a life-threatening health issue. Or you wake up in the middle of the night to give permission for a parent to be given shock treatment by the EMS or you receive a call from the Emergency Room. You may even be in another State at the time!

Sometimes life moves slowly, and time allows for gradual change as a person ages and realizes help is needed with daily life tasks. Other times you run into a brick wall at full speed when a loved one has been diagnosed with cancer, Parkinsons, Lewey Body type disease or has had a stroke. Change and obligation could simply happen after the fact of any emergency hospital visit when sitting at the discharge desk with a kind paper-pushing discharge person saying "Here is the discharge notes, follow up with primary physician within blah blah days, let us know if blah-blah happens, here is the prescription to add to the current medication, let us know if there are any reactions, make sure to take blah-blah, wha-wha-wha... and the co-pay is $$$, how do you want to pay?" As you sit there with a deer-in-the-headlight look on your face, reeling with emotions and see to do lists dancing in your head, you begin to feel dizzy. Then the light bulb goes off, how will I take care of all this, work, take care of the rest of my family and make sure all the bills will get paid?

Any of these situations is an entry into what I have labeled "The Gauntlet of Caregiving."

When I was a child, we had telephones instead of iPhones or Androids. These shapely hunks of plastic either sat on table, kitchen counter or resided in a fancy designed telephone nook. Some were mounted on the wall with long cords to give more mobility while talking. It seemed like every funeral home had the same marketing company, because every elderly adult had a funeral home sticker plastered across the handle of the phone! Basic emergency numbers such as Police, fire department, ambulance, doctor name and number were easily accessible by anyone using the telephone. No question where to go to find this information. An amazing common thread throughout every city and State across America. Truly a phenomenal societal connection if you think about it. So simple, a sticker on every telephone in America. Added to this was the telephone directory delivered to every person who had a telephone. The very first page, inside cover was a blank chart where the resident could write a list of important contacts including addresses and phone numbers in case of emergency.

Noting this amazing tradition has disappeared, it begs for a new solution and brings this question to mind. How would someone find out just one piece of important information like this about you or your Loved One today?

By the time you finish reading the many or selected sections of this book, my hope is you will have a clearer vision of how to answer this question and many others that will not be known until they arise. It is surprising the assumptions we make about our Loved One's personal lives; the goal of this whole project is to help anyone be more prepared to help your family when the need arises. An even better outcome would be having everything prepared prior to this need on your part.

I do not believe the average person is prepared emotionally, physically, or financially for a loved one who becomes extremely ill or incapacitated. Often with parents the decline is gradual, and we are lovingly dutiful to help. But there will come a time when being a full-time caregiver is needed and it can be overwhelming whether it is gradual or an acute need that arises.

On the surface of a tragedy, everyone sees and provides emotional support to the caregiver. Behind the scenes loved ones and most of all the caregivers, often and out of necessity, treat their own emotions like the elephant in the corner that no one wants to talk about. Why? Because once you enter "The Gauntlet of Caregiving" and the complete and total care of someone else, the focus becomes how to survive the system, make sure your loved one is actually being taken care of (by you or someone else) and make sure the bills will be paid. And then there are family dynamics that add to the situation. Family relationships will not be covered in this book, but the content is designed to help offset and avoid many issues.

The many hats of caregiving will cause your hair to wear thin. At any given time you are expected to not only know how to fit into a specific role, but have complete knowledge, efficient implementation ability, precision communication systems in place, and, among so many other skills, provide twenty-four-seven culinary, housekeeping, transportation, nursing, accounting, legal and mental health support to another human being.

This is the reality folks.

I ask you to Hang on to your sense of humor, dig deep into your numb emotional suitcase and prepare to enter The Gauntlet. Be prepared to be prepared and successful!

Who does what for whom?

To get started, the most unanswered question about the definition of caregiver is who does what in the realm of caregiving for someone else?

Let's start by dissecting the concept of being a caregiver. This catchall word actually describes the duty of taking care of another person. There are volumes of books and writings about caregiving too extensive to enumerate in this book. But as a whole the healthcare industry has expanded into an all-encompassing lifestyle of caregiving options as you will read about in Chapter 8. Here is a brief description obtained over time, by many sources, including experience, which describe a caregiver.

Caregiver: A person who gives care to another person usually in their home performing duties of daily life such as helping with housekeeping, running errands, cooking, and other duties. A caregiver can be hired, be a family member or friend. Understanding what services a person needs can be a gradual process of seeing what is needed or having the needs evaluated by a professional.

Primary Caregiver: A person who may give daily life care or may not. The primary caregiver may be the "Captain of the Ship" leading a team of what is sometimes termed secondary caregivers. The responsibilities can include what was stated in the previous paragraph as well as being power of attorney, named in advance directives or medical power of attorney, agent of a living will or participant in the last will and testament. The primary caregiver may be named as guardian or conservator. Each State has statutes and/or legal definitions for these roles and some government entity may offer compensation for caregiving roles at home as well.

When does a Primary Caregiver become viable? From a caregiving perspective, as soon as someone begins needing help. Whether to organize daily assistance, handle finances, or healthcare, the time can come suddenly or gradually. The need for a primary caregiver to implement the authority given to them by a Power of Attorney or Healthcare directive is often considered subjective. Therefore consultation with an attorney when documents are signed, and documentation of acts performed is paramount. As always, the best practice is defaulting and including the person in your care when making life decisions. This process can also be helpful when there are many family members and only one person is given the task as primary caregiver.

For ease of writing, the word "caregiver" will be used as the general term for both of these roles. Many forms will be assigned to another or many other caregivers. Do not take the roles as literally separated or together! Make sure there is a "Primary Caregiver" otherwise the task of giving care can become not only confusing but also dangerous for the person who needs care.

There are some legal guidelines in Chapter 7 about the legal responsibilities regarding the acceptance of being a primary caregiver. Be cautious and know what you are signing up to do.

What is the difference between a conservator or guardian and a primary caregiver?

It is best to consult an attorney to define the differences within the State where someone has domicile. In general a conservator or guardian are appointed by a court. Sometimes a guardian is used for a person who is a child, and a conservator is used for an adult. Their duties can include financial and healthcare duties for someone unable to do it for themselves. It all depends on the legal statutes in a State.

A primary caregiver is designated by a person needing care and the supporting documentation gives them specific permissions regarding daily life decisions.

What is the difference between a primary caregiver and an executor of an estate?

The primary caregiver: handles the daily life of someone during their living years.

The executor or trustee: of an estate will handle affairs after death.

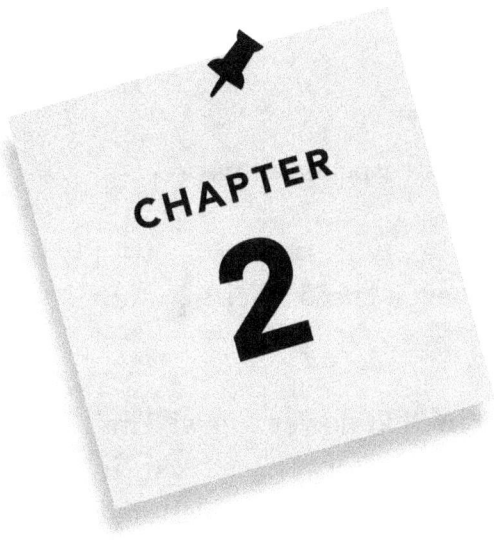

CHAPTER

2

Orderly Reading – Why?

Why not!

This chapter represents the information contained within the Gauntlet and is presented in an order of what the author believes is important. Yet, for like-minded individuals the author also believes that there are times when random access to information is paramount especially when an unforeseen situation arises, or just because you can.

By Design.
This book has been created in a large format for ease of use. Please earmark pages, write notes, place sticky notes, so you can use in the way that works best for you.

The Essential Information List, Chapter 3.
The Essentials list is what everyone needs to gather together in order to have someone else take care of their needs. If you are a caregiver and have not been provided with this information it will be helpful for everyone if this information is collected, once done, you can help accomplish this task. There is an example of this form in the Appendix of this book. You can use this list to collect the information, type your own or order a preprinted bundle, ready to use package from the same vendor you used to purchase this book.

The Emotional Gauntlet of Merging Lifestyles, Chapter 4.
If you have ever had a roommate, this will bring back memories! Please read this chapter. It will help to understand why you, as a caregiver, need respite care which is described in Chapter 9.

The Data Dump Gauntlet, Chapter 5.
There are three parts to this chapter. Each is distinctly different aspects of this process, yet all are linked together for a cohesive care plan.

Part 1; learning to communicate while assessing daily routines and needs. Getting away from the clinical questioning side of caregiving.

Part 2; getting to know the person you may think you know, but do you know? This chapter helps to give new insight into the real person and their history instead of their forever role in a family. This history will help to fill in questions on the "Personal Information" form which is essential for helping to fill out healthcare information at healthcare facilities.

Part 3; the details of the data dump. Yes, this is a very straightforward question and answer session to help fill in the blanks of the "Personal Information" form. These questions are very personal and following the steps in Parts 1 & 2 will help you, the caregiver, to be looked on as a person who cares rather than a person who is just asking lots of personal questions. If the person who is being cared for has already filled out their information forms, fantastic! Be sure to date the top to know when it was last updated. This will provide a baseline for future healthcare documentation. Once a healthcare change happens updates should be made and dated.

The Healthcare Management Gauntlet, Chapter 6.
A discussion about advocates. Just when you believe someone can answer all of your questions, you are left alone again. The healthcare advocate: what they are, what they are not, and what to expect from them.

The Legal Gauntlet, Chapter 7.
This chapter is divided into three parts. Each section provides different aspects of the legalese encountered in different situations of taking care of someone else's affairs.

The Gauntlet of Congregate Living, Chapter 8.
This chapter will define and introduce you to the realty vs myths of alternative housing.

The Respite Gauntlets, Chapter 9.
This chapter introduces you, the caregiver, to the pitfalls of being a full-time and part-time caregiver and an in-depth discussion about the need for respite care and why. There are also suggestions for finding a temporary replacement for yourself in order to set time aside for respite care.

The Gauntlet of Medication Management, Chapter 10.
Medications and their management are one of the most important daily life tasks to plan for and execute. There are many levels of medication management and the options to accomplish this task are many.

How To Organize Everyday Paperwork, Chapter 11.
This three-part chapter is a must read. It will help organize the everyday communication between caregiving team members. Whether a team of one or of m-a-n-y easily accessing records will make being a caregiver less stressful. This organization setup includes everything from daily living habits, appointments, health records, health information to financial records and final arrangements. This book is the treasure map to documents wherever they may be hiding whether a box, file cabinet, safe or with someone else. Using this easy-to-follow system there will no longer be any guesswork to find any vital records.

Binders and Such, Chapter 12.
Here you will find reviews for what the author has stumbled through over time to help organize daily life for the caregiver and the person being cared for. Also, at a future date there will be an option to purchase the system online and ready to go.

Organizational Notebook Downloads, Chapter 13.
This section gives links to access and download all the forms in PDF format to organize the notebooks. A packet of pre-printed forms can be ordered. Examples of the forms are also included in the Appendix of this book.

Resources, Chapter 14.
This section has important information about organizations that can provide specific care guidelines for specific states. For example, healthcare directives are legally different in each state, Medicaid options and other services are also different depending on the state of residence.

If you wish to share something you have discovered while caregiving, please email the author at info.gauntletofcaregiving@gmail.com.

What this book is and is not.
This book does not go into details about some caregiving subjects such as daily care giving duties regarding hygiene, dietary care, physical or occupational therapies, etc. Neither does it cover caring for disabled children. This is a very specific need which the

author has a familiarity with through working at a not-for-profit company but believes it is best left to the professionals for health and legal guidance on this matter.

What this book is focused on is providing a way to manage care. We live in a managed care society. Every institution has a charting system. For someone being cared for at home, this book will guide you through creating a managed care and life care charting system to be used across all of the gauntlet of services needed by an individual who can no longer do it themselves.

CHAPTER

3

The Essential Information List

First things first!

Before we begin gathering the essential information, decisions must be made regarding who will be the "Primary Caregiver." If you have not read Chapter 1, please return there and read about the difference between a "Caregiver" and a "Primary Caregiver." Then move on to read about the Legal Gauntlet in Chapter 7. Legal mistakes are often made unintentionally out of a heartfelt interest to help someone.

Important Personal Information

To the person needing care. This information and its location should be readily available to the person who will be a caregiver if ever needed. Whether a Spouse, Child, Relative or Friend, it is imperative that someone has access so that YOU can be taken care of when needed.

If there is a confidence or conflict issue, a third party such as an Attorney, Conservator or Guardian should be assigned to hold this information.

Identification requirements

- Driver's License(s) or State Issued ID
- Social Security Card(s)
- Birth Certificate
- Proof of Citizenship or Green card

- Passport
- Veteran: DD214 (As of 2024)
- Pension Identification Card(s)

Personal Health Information*

- Medicare Card(s)
- Supplemental Health Insurance Cards (Copy front & back)
- Long Term Health Care Insurance
- Dental & Vision Insurance
- Other Health Plans such as VA, Government Employee, or Pension Plans (Do not copy Government ID's especially Military ID's, it is a violation and illegal)
- List of Current Medications, Prescribing Doctor, Use & Dosage (Health History Form)
- List of Current Doctors or Specialty Care Physician(s) (Health History Form)
- List of Doctors Recently Scene in Hospital (Health History Form)
- Health History (Health History Form)
- Living Will (See Links to State Requirements)
- Healthcare Directive (See Links to State Requirements)
- Healthcare Surrogate Designation (See Links to State Requirements)
- Healthcare Power of Attorney (See Links to State Requirements)

Personal Assets and Financial Management*

- Motor Vehicle Registration or Title (Cars, Campers, Motorcycle, Mobile Homes) If financed, Financial Institution information, copy of loan(s) & Payment Information
- Income Verification from ALL sources including Pension Benefits
- Checking/Savings, Brokerage accounts, Statements of all for past 3-6 months
- Income Tax Filing for last 5 yrs.
- Mortgage Information (Asset Liability Form)
- Property Tax Bill(s) & Addresses (The property address does not always appear on the bill)
- Property Insurance Providers (Homeowners, Vehicle, Boat, Camper, Golf Cart, Motorcycle, etc.)
- Personal Residence and Value (Required for Government programs that are based on assets and income such as Medicaid, County/City in Home Care, & other programs)

- Technology Usernames and Passwords for online accounts. (NOTE: Companies will not allow anyone other than an authorized user to talk about an account. Not even the cable, cell phone or water company. Either the owner must provide permission each time or a POA must be on file in order to take care of services.)
- Power of Attorney (Durable and/or stated powers) There could be multiple people with POA's performing different duties on someone's behalf. These should all be included! Do not assume to perform any legal act or transaction on the behalf of someone else without knowing what is in writing. Never assume!

Legal and Professional*

- Long-Term Care Insurance Policies
- Business Papers: Partnership Agreements, Financial Statements, Buy/Sell Agreements
- Life Insurance and Annuity Policies including current values.
- Funeral Planning Declaration (Include all Details)
- Trust Agreements or TOD – Transfer on Death Deed for Real Estate
- Last Will and Testament (Attorney Name or Where is it held)
- Estate Planning and/or Elder Care Attorney Name and Contact Information

Takeaways:

- For an explanation of these items refer to Chapter 11. "How To Organize Everyday Paperwork" Part 1, 2 and 3.
- An example of this list can be seen in the Appendix. It will be included in the packet of forms which can be ordered separately.

CHAPTER

4

Emotional Gauntlet of Merging Lifestyles

Do You Really Know Your Loved One?

On a rare occasion when I accompanied Mom to the doctor, I was enlightened by how much paperwork was required for a regular patient. She had always been fiercely independent, so she insisted on filling in the blanks on her own. I was feeling completely out of my element!

During one occasion as she filled out the paperwork, she looked at me and said "this question is odd… 'Did you have trouble sleeping as a child?' Should I answer yes, and say because of bombing?" We both had a good laugh. Mom was born and raised in England, a part of Great Britain. She came to America at the age of twenty-one. When she was around 7 years of age World War II began, the year was 1940 when the German Nazis began bombing missions over England.

Laughter was something that Mom believed in. When all else looks bleak, the soul often reaches a point when it becomes too numb to feel. Laughter can bring in a fresh new perspective and connection. I knew she had been exposed to many horrific situations, but I had given little thought to how it had influenced her in every aspect of her everyday life. We live in America after all and since the 1960's life has been pretty consistent, well except for the Pandemic in 2020 and shortages of items like toilet paper in 2022. Living with bombings, displacement and rationing of everything including food can certainly influence a person's outlook and behavior. Tenacity is what she called her perseverance.

I do not share these experiences to cause divisiveness. History is not meant for that purpose. It educates us as humans with several outcomes, but not hate, revenge, or discrimination. History opens our eyes and our minds to the capabilities of human frailty which can manifest in many ways when the need to survive, thrive and satisfy a basic need has been shattered. Mom taught me this.

> *If you have read to this point, take a break, do something good for yourself. Just being here is a part of the emotional gauntlet.*
>
> *Also, there is an explanation later on why technology isn't recommended, and the organizational notebooks fill a much-needed niche for the role of caregiver.*

Old Words of Wisdom and Generational Caregiving

As it has been said by many who know Christian scripture, Cain killed Abel with a rock. David killed Goliath with a rock. Each tool took someone's life. One was considered by God as a sin. The other is an act of self-defense. This difference is why we have laws and the justice system as declared by the American forefathers. So far history has shown that our justice system has been the best answer, even though it is not without flaws.

I mention words of wisdom along with history, law, and differences in this section because it is not only important to understand the world that has influenced the person you care for, but also you as a caregiver. This is a particularly important aspect of generational caregiving, whether the person is a peer, older or younger. Just like the everlasting debate about which way the toilet paper is placed on the holder, there comes a time when a decision must be made. As a caregiver, our views on the world and everyday activities must move to the background. Your opinion of how the toilet paper should be stored should be set aside. If you do not agree, that is ok. But consider this. If someone walked into your home, declared you unable to be independent and took over all aspects of your life, what would you expect? If it meant giving no consideration to who you are, what your beliefs are, what your history and experience has been in life, how would you feel? Considering the one you care for while providing a dignified environment is paramount. Leaving your own goals, sensitivities and emotions at the door unfortunately is a part of caregiving. This is one of the biggest challenges, the "Emotional Gauntlet of Merging Lifestyles."

Know the Person You are Caring For

To be an effective caregiver, you must know as much as possible about the person you are caring for. Just saying, Oh, he is my Dad, or Mom or Brother does not mean you know that person. Knowing my mother as well as I did was helpful. But there was so much that was still unknown. What was her daily routine, did she have one? Yes. Finding out what that routine entailed was a challenge. I knew she called me regularly these days about 3:00, she was social, she drank hot tea, enjoyed dancing, she loved to laugh, and she set high standards for character. What else could there be to know?

So often we adapt when people come to visit, routines change and then if visitors stay long enough, they will experience daily life revert back to a different pace. For example, the saying "Company, like fish, begins to be unwelcome after three days." There is much truth in the saying for many reasons. What this means too is that when you visit someone, even family, the hosting member often bypasses normal routines to accommodate the visitor. This deviation is only comfortable for a short time. Then it is important for the hosting family member to re-establish a more normal routine. For example, the full breakfast that was served every morning turns into help yourself cereal. After a short period of time, the host begins to do their own thing and possibly distance themselves from the visitors. So, will it happen in caregiving? More than likely, it will, and this is when feelings get hurt. This conflict is one of the most common issues I have experienced and been told about when caring for someone else. No matter if the caregiver is a close relative that is well known as a parent or even a spouse or a friend.

Caregiver Conflicts

Here are some common conflicts to which you may relate. Some I have experienced, and others have been shared with me by others. Be forewarned, you will see the personal pronoun "I" often in the following list.

- I eat breakfast at 9:00 am. Why do I have to eat at 8:00?

- Write it on the calendar. I will look at the calendar. I do not want a smart phone.

- I want my meds in my little pill box. That is what I know. Do not tell me when to take them, I have my routine.

- When are you leaving? I want to do things the way I do them.

- Why do I have to shower so often? Do not tell me when I need to shower. Do not tell me what I need to do.

- That helper doesn't dust or clean the way I do.

- I use the dishwasher to store clean dishes.

- Why are the wrong color towels in the bathroom?

- Why can't I get my TV program? Why did we change cable companies? What is streaming? I want my channels back!

- I don't want to draw. I have never drawn stuff! Crayons are for kids!

- Why did I have to move? The closet isn't right or too small or too different.

- Don't talk to me like a child. I fought in the war. (This one can be multi generation and spans past wars from WWII to Afghanistan and beyond.)

- I bowl every Wednesday in the league. Why did the doctor say I can't drive?

- Why are you looking through my mail?

- Why do you want my banking information?

- You do things your way. I do things my way.

And so many more. Often these issues come up because the caregiver needs to set a routine that is in keeping with his/her own world. Often the first complaint that is expressed by a Caregiver is "I do all this for them, and all I hear are complaints, or that something isn't right…"

For everyone's sanity getting to know the other person's lifestyle and routines can help everyone be less stressed by this emotional gauntlet.

Being organized in other areas, in your own way as a Caregiver, will empower you to deal with the emotional gauntlet in a more confident, less stressful way. Using this book to create a system and knowing you can access information needed for the multiple calls, appointments, forms, likes, dislikes, and endless communications needed by every entity known on the planet, will help everyone to successfully navigate through this new daily life.

Takeaways:

- Plan conversation time. Get to know the person you are caring for. A list of prepared questions about likes, habits, routines, etc. that will encourage dialog can be found in Chapter 5.
- Take a look at "How to Organize Everyday Paperwork" Chapter 11, to get started sorting the mountain of legal, accounting, healthcare, and personal information paperwork that is important for current needs.

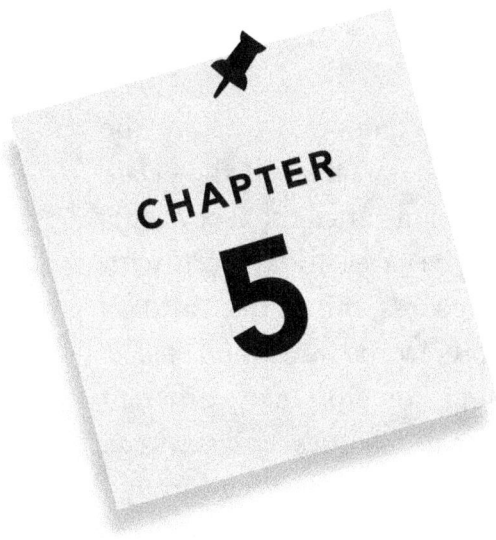

CHAPTER

5

The Data Dump
Gauntlet – Part 1

Gathering Information

This section is divided into three parts. Part 1 is to help the Caregiver focus on getting to know the schedules, daily routines, and dietary needs of the person to whom they are giving care.

Part 2 is directed toward getting to know the person you are taking care of. It also will bring forth life stories that can help with gathering family, healthcare, and other historic data. Why you may ask, well, do you remember having your tonsils removed at age 3 or having tubes in your ears at age 1? If you do, fantastic. How many other people know?

Part 3 discusses the reason for the need to complete the data sheets and how to meet healthcare information requirements at doctor office visits, emergency care or hospital admissions. All parts are paramount in order to have a complete understanding of what is necessary to confidently fulfill the role of Caregiver.

Once you are involved with caregiving, there are processes with questionnaires that are presented in obnoxious and repetitive manners. Data collection without consideration that a real person is answering and not an artificial intelligence apparatus can be impersonal and upsetting to a healthy person, and more so to someone who is aged, ill or disabled. As a caregiver, having information and being able to fill in the blanks to help can be a great stress reliever.

These questions and examples are for those who are lucky enough to have the opportunity to communicate with the person who is the main target of the "Data Dump Gauntlet." As the caregiver, taking on the repercussions after the fact of this gauntlet is much more difficult. Why may you ask? To be brief, today even with technology, there is not a complete system for healthcare records. It is unlike the days when a person had one doctor in one office and all medical records were in one place. Today this healthcare information is fractured and is being stored on many different portals, hard drives, mobile devices, or in boxes in storage facilities or elsewhere. Being prepared and pro-active by collecting information will help to proceed through the myriad of questionnaires, forms and processes required by healthcare providers, bankers, accountants, government agencies, and countless others. Also, when a discrepancy occurs between what a patient hears and what a healthcare provider says, documentation can prove to be lifesaving.

The common data collecting barrage of questions, line after line, page after page, person after person, can make anyone feel overwhelmed and unimportant. This phenomenon reminds this author of the verse in a Pink Floyd tune, 'just another brick in the wall' from the song of the same name… "Another Brick in the Wall." What is important is that you, as a caregiver, become as confident as possible with current information and not be stuck in a situation that is without a solution.

Along with getting to know the person you are caring for, completing the Personal Health Information form, and including it in the white "Organizational Notebook," will help avoid the stressful events experienced by the "Data Dump Gauntlet." This form will provide the data needed to complete the plethora of information forms required by healthcare institutions.

Using the following questions may seem silly or elementary, but it is the little things in daily life that are considered certainties and create an environment of stability. Collecting the answers to these questions and adding the information to your appropriate Daily Activities and Healthcare Organizational Notebooks will help greatly. Try it and take notes of the answers. They will come in handy!

A Digressive Explanation

Each question in Part 1 and Part 2 has a brief explanation that will help you ease into finding out information. Keeping questions in a conversational realm will help to offset the "Data Dump Gauntlet" feeling. By incorporating these questions into easy conversations, they will also lead to many useful and interesting discoveries!

A "Mom Taught Me Moment": War or upheaval of routines and certainties can create chaos and insecurity. Mom told me she survived because "my girlfriends and I planned to meet and go dancing. It gave us focus, something we knew we could look forward to as a routine, something on which we could depend. We went to the same dance hall, we walked together, laughed, and chatted about silly, nonsensical things. A way to escape the reality of bombings, death, and fear."

Let's get on and start with those silly, seemingly elementary questions that will help to fill in the blanks on the "Daily Routine" forms in the "Daily Organizational Notebook" (Purple book as recommended in Chapter 11, How To Organize Everyday Paperwork).

- What do you like to drink?

- How do you make your coffee or tea?

- What brand or type of coffee/tea do you like?

- How many scoops of coffee makes a good cup?

- How much milk or creamer do you add to make a good cup?

- Do you use bottled or tap water to make your coffee?

If the answer is short, such as "Black," or I do not drink coffee, move on, you can briefly tell them how you do yours. Also, when they wrinkle their nose at your coffee, it is a sign to ask more questions and do not talk about yourself! If no more information is forthcoming, move on to the other questions. Make notes if needed to make sure he/she knows you want to do it their way.

I think about Jeremy Clarkson on "Clarkson's Farm" TV series when he expressed at the end of a rather difficult and stressful day, he needed a "cuppa tea" hot, sweet, and milky, to make it all better. He surely has access to any beverage he would like. Now we know what helps him relax!

A one-sided conversation like the following can sometimes give the impression you like to talk about yourself rather than his/her needs. Ask me how I know…

"I make my coffee one cup at a time with a Keurig machine, decaf only. I fill the reservoir with bottled water, pop a pod of my favorite coffee in the machine, and brew.

I then heat the milk in my frothier and pour the hot steamy milk into my cup, adding a teaspoon of raw sugar."

It is difficult to sometimes fill in the silent, awkward space in a conversation with chatter, but often someone who needs care, whether knowingly or subconsciously, wants to be the caregivers' only focus. Believe me, this is true!

Laundry Schedule. Is there such a thing? How to find out how idiosyncratic people can be, just ask how they like their laundry done. Really.

Add these notes to the purple "Daily Activities Organizational Notebook."

- Do you wash your sheets on a specific day?

- Which do you prefer to use, fabric softener in the wash or fabric softener sheets in the dryer?

- What kind of laundry detergent do you like?

Having listened to others talk about this subject has made me realize how important the answers to daily living questions truly are. Some people do NOT want softener sheets in the dryer, or just want them for clothing and not towels or sheets. Then again, liquid softener could be preferred for all the laundry.

The brands are important also because smell is one of our highest-ranking senses. It can stamp the brain with a situation, place, date, or person. The use of other brands or options may create an environment for personal sensitivities. Even the smell of food cooked with a different oil can trigger an emotional reaction. I have seen this often.

The movie "Saving Private Ryan" is a good example of how emotional recall can be triggered. I read somewhere about an interview that stated when the movie was previewed by WWII Veterans, they were asked questions afterwards. One question included this; "how real and accurate was its content." (FYI, I paraphrase) A common answer was, "it had everything but the smell…"

- What do you usually eat for breakfast?

- What is your favorite meal for lunch?

- What time do you like to eat (breakfast, lunch, dinner)?

- What do you like to eat for dinner?

- Do you snack between meals? (If so, what is your favorite snack?)

- Do you like vegetables? Fruit? How do you like them prepared?

- Do you like dessert with dinner? What is your favorite?

Breakfast is an important meal according to most information provided by the healthcare industry about nutrition. Having spoken with professional nutritionists when caregiving, it makes sense after basically fasting for hours when sleeping (6-8 usually, if lucky) the body wakes up and is ready for some kind of supplement. This meal must meet any dietary constraint recommendations of the healthcare provider and should be noted as a question to ask on the next visit with the physician. Often a loved one has settled into a routine of some sort. If a change has been made to a person's diet, it should be noted in the most recent doctor's office visit notes. The "Daily Routine Form" can help organize and record daily dietary needs.

When you and your friends go to (the Club, meeting, Church service or social), what do you do there?

- Do you usually have a meal or snacks? Did you like what was served?

- What kind of food do you prefer to eat when you go out to a restaurant?

- Have you been anywhere that you didn't like the food that was provided?

This is a basic conversation starter for sure. The result can be incredibly sad, happy, or even enlightening with a result that will help the caregiver become aware of the type of foods that are appealing or that are distasteful. The statement 'sad' means that what may have been a favorite dish at one time may no longer be enjoyed. There are many causes for this and are often due to medications taken, dietary restrictions or other health issues that have affected taste. Even the ability to chew or swallow can restrict food consumption that was once favorites.

Another informative bit is about people who prefer to do the cooking. Often anyone else who has prepared food comes under great scrutiny. Many times, stories have been relayed that caregivers see this kind of 'no one cooks like me attitude' which can often lead to a reduced appetite. This situation could be dangerous and should be noted by date, time, reaction, type of food, etc. so the caregiver can track and inform the doctor or other healthcare professionals.

Social Activities

- What activities did you enjoy at (the Club, meeting, Church service or social)

- What is your favorite activity?

- How often do you participate in the activity (playing cards, chorus, golfing)?

- Would you like to do it more often? (This question should let you know if it is still a viable activity or how long it has been since the activity was done)

Many people enjoy social events. It is healthy for people to mingle and engage socially. But if someone has been a loner most of their life or possibly has changed in a disabling way, expecting them to welcome busy social situations can have consequences. The results will depend on the caregivers' ability to know when to encourage connection or exit gracefully.

Another important aspect of asking about social gatherings is that often more history about a person is revealed. For example, if the meetings or socializing was at the VFW, a history of military and possible service colleagues is discovered. These friendships are so important to maintain when possible and you, the caregiver, become the conduit for continued connections. This information would also mean that possible healthcare was done or is done through the Veterans Administration.

There is a place to list contacts for friends that may enjoy visiting. This list can be made on the "About Us & Our Home" form found in the purple "Daily Activities" notebook. Often these people may be members of a club, organization or other activity and contact can be a very welcome break and emotional boost from daily monotony due to changes in someone's health status.

Takeaways:

- Getting to know the person you are caring for is paramount! Even if that person is a parent, you may think you know them intimately. But you will be surprised at how little you know about them as an individual until the need for caregiving arises and you start to ask questions.
- There is a list of Important Information questions that are absolutely necessary to have answered as a caregiver, use the "Important Personal and Health Information" form, the "Healthcare Provider Appointment Notes" and "Daily Routine" Form. These should be included in the (Purple) "Organizational Paperwork" Daily Activity notebook.
- As a caregiver, be prepared to take care of yourself. See Chapter 9, The Respite Care Gauntlet.

The Data Dump Gauntlet - Part 2
Getting To Know Someone You Already Know?

Before my Daughter-in-law had her disabling stroke, she was continually active and loved to bowl on a League. When her stroke happened, her team had just won the Championship Competition. While she was still in the hospital truly fighting for her life, the team shared a picture of her taken with the team and the trophy. I knew she bowled as a hobby but had no idea she was so good!

It took time for me to recognize that my daughter-in-law enjoys crafts and can do them with her disability. So, when I am at her home to give my son respite times, having a craft is a wonderful engaging and fun thing to do together.

The Embarrassment Gauntlet:

Regarding family, especially parents and children. Life happens and often we do not recognize that a person in a certain role, such as a parent, is not looked on as an individual. What does this mean? It means how do you see that person, is it the same way you see a friend? Think about it, would you assume that when helping a friend you would go into their home and rearrange everything to suit your comfort? Would you tell a friend they should arrange their house a certain way, or do things the right way (which is your way)? This happens so often with spouses, siblings, relatives, and aging parents. It is a phenomenon that is assumed to be ok. But to help make life easier as a caregiver the goal is not to change someone else's life to make yours easier. It is to get to know the person you care for in order to help them be as comfortable as possible and live in a dignified way while you help them. Discovering this lack of awareness prior to the point of becoming a caregiver can be overwhelming, but you have got this. Take a deep breath, the only person who knows you may be embarrassed is you.

You may think, why bother reading on?

Even though this section may seem silly, going through this process will not only be helpful to you as a Caregiver, but you may learn something about someone you never knew before! This knowledge may also touch your heart in ways that encourage you to share with someone else. Sometimes this opportunity creates a legacy from one person to another. There is a particularly good possibility the person you believed you knew has had a life never revealed before.

Getting To Know Someone Questions

- Of all the places you have visited, which do you recall enjoying the most?

- Do you have pictures of places you have visited?

- Did you collect mementos from the places you visited?

- Which place did you enjoy the least?

- Is there a special reason you did not like that place or the visit?

Yes, not all questions should only focus on positive memories. Learning how a person remembers how discomforting it was to not find the bathroom in a country that has no English signage is important! Just as important as that fabulous little café on a quaint street in Paris that served the flakiest croissants ever. Bingo. A comfort food and knowing a bathroom break being convenient can make a person's day brighter. Good lessons!

- When you work(ed), what do you enjoy doing the most?

- When you work(ed), which task do you enjoy the least?

- What exactly is/was your job?

Have you had more than one career?

Years ago, I worked in a retirement center. We had Independent, Assisted Living, Acute Care and Long-Term Care facilities all on the same campus. I worked in Administration. There was a resident that always came into our office to consult with the Executive Director about the day-to-day operations. He would stop by on his walk over to the Assisted Living building where his wife was residing, while he remained in Independent Living, a perfect setup for them. He remained a highly active and agile gentleman. I really enjoyed our interactions when there was an opportunity to speak.

I never asked about his life. I was young and had hopes of moving up the career ladder, not understanding the life stories our residents brought with them. When he passed, I asked what he had done for a living. To my shock, he had been a senior editor at Life Magazine. Oh, what a life he had had. Having asked the right questions, I could have learned so much about him and the world he had lived in.

- Here are some fun questions.

- Have you ever jumped out of a plane, (with a parachute, of course)?

- Have you ever gone white-water rafting?

- Have you ever driven a racecar?

- Have you ever skied on snow or water?

- Have you ever flown in a plane or been a pilot?

- Have you hiked a mountain?

The first question is one of my personal favorites. It usually gets a laugh, but it can start some amazing conversations, often leading to more laughter and sometimes amazing stories as well as personal history.

My favorite uncle was such a great communicator. As rarely as we visited face to face, he would always teach me something about myself and give me a little peek deeper into my father's side of the family. On one occasion, he asked me if I had heard of the island Tinian. Replying like a typical young person, I answered nope. So, he proceeded to tell me the story of how he was on the island of Tinian during WWII with the infamous Enola Gay. (Here is your chance to use a search engine.) He was a radio technician on one of four B-29's running missions from the island, when his plane crashed. As a radio guy, his seat was at the bottom of the plane. He happened to be located elsewhere when the crash occurred which saved his life. A chilling story for the listener, but the way he told it was humble and humorous.

So, I always expect the unexpected when using the question about jumping out of an airplane. My answer to that question is yes, I have; for the fun of it!

- Do you have a favorite pillow? Is it a feather pillow or other material?

- Do you have a favorite shampoo? What is your brand?

- Do you use liquid shower soap or bar soap to bathe? What brand?

- Do you use the dishwasher or wash the dishes by hand?

- What kind of dishwashing soap do you use?

These random questions have been extremely helpful in discovering several things of importance. Especially for someone who is ill, had a stroke or suffers from some type of issue such as waking up at intervals during the night instead of staying asleep. When someone must go to a hospital, a rehab facility or have a hospital bed installed in their home, the right pillow can be a comfort or a nemesis, no matter the age. A favorite brand of soap or shampoo can give a feeling of comfort and familiarity. For someone who has served in the military, some smells can bring back bad or good memories as well.

The information gathered through these kinds of conversations can also help when filling out the personal information pages. Often when asking data questions an ill or aging person may forget he/she had a wound or had pins put in to repair a broken bone. It is amazing what can be forgotten at any age. Revisiting experiences can bring forth a plethora of important information. Once written down, you have it!

There are so many more questions, write them down here in the margins and if you are inclined to share yours, suggestions are always welcomed. It would be my pleasure to include them as an added section.

Takeaways:

- Part 2 of the "Data Dump Gauntlet" is as important as Part 1 and 3.
- Organizational Paperwork Note Page Forms will help to categorize notes for healthcare visits.
- Organizational Paperwork Daily Routine Forms will keep dietary and daily routines easily accessible.

The Data Dump Gauntlet - Part 3

We are a Data Driven Society…

Have you ever thought about how much information you keep in your brain or on your smartphone? The amount of information stored that no one else has access to is overwhelming if you actually stop and think about it. At any time have you shared any of this personal health or family history information with someone? Well, welcome to the reality of the "Data Dump Gauntlet" of Healthcare and Legal information.

If you were in a car accident and became unconscious, who would know anything about you other than what your ID says? Most people carry basic information in a wallet or purse, sometimes a cell phone will have emergency contacts, but who will actually know your wishes regarding care if you are not able to speak for yourself. The answer is yes, we all would hope that whoever is in charge, whether a loved one or a healthcare provider, would do the absolute best to get you back into a healthy state.

The fear of the unknown is what insurance companies, attorneys, and many other corporations hope will happen so that you will purchase a plan for the unknown future. This book is not to persuade you to do that. This journey of reading is to provide a basic awareness of what it is like for a person who, right now, needs a caregiver to take care of them in a way that provides dignity, safety, and consistency, whether they have prepared for this time or not.

So how can you help yourself or someone else? This is where the Data Dump Gauntlet becomes strictly informational. Boring, yes, necessary, yes! This section is so basic that many times it is overlooked by everyone. Objections to sharing this personal information can result in frustration when the time comes to help as a caregiver or be helped.

What is required by healthcare professionals is no less than a dissertation on how to limit their liability, justify the treatment to a patient, to stay within the Health Insurance Portability and Accountability Act (HIPAA) law to protect patient information, while getting paid by insurance carriers, and prevent frivolous malpractice lawsuits. This long sentence describes the many facets of managed care that came into being in the 1980's when DRG's (diagnosis-related group) became the measurement of good healthcare. And in 1996 HIPAA created the sharing of information legal bottleneck.

This statement is not meant to blame anyone, but to point out that a caregiver having complete health information is paramount to facilitate the evaluation of a person's healthcare and fulfill a healthcare and daily life plan that will work best for them. As a caregiver you have the best chance to have the most comprehensive information collected by filling out the data needed on the Personal Information form, which is extensive. It will come in handy to review when needing to fill out endless different questionnaires at healthcare facilities and physicians' offices. It is sometimes surprising how many different places a patient will be sent when a health issue arises. There used to be the option to have everything from x-rays to blood work done in a physician's office and stored locally when access was needed. These days it is all at different locations and often stored virtually. HIPAA (Health Insurance Portability and Accountability Act) requires compliant portals for health information storage. It seems every healthcare provider uses a different source for this storage and there are required usernames and passwords for everyone, over time this can become a huge imposition just to remember the names of portals, how to access and what doctor the information was connected with. Also there is the issue of internet connection. No connection, no access to records.

Why are paper notebooks necessary? I was blessed with caregiving for a friend of ninety plus years, he was a highly organized individual. Because he insisted on knowing who was coming, what service was being provided, when it was to be accomplished, he insisted on having things written down. So, my organization skills began to develop. He expected everyone to know this information. My caregiving responsibilities became making sure communication between outside caregivers, home visit Physicians, outside healthcare providers, independent living administrators, food service providers in house and outsourced, were all able to know what was going on, who was scheduled, what was scheduled, how things were scheduled as well as how the daily life of the person/patient was going. Every aspect of daily living was logged, confirmed, tangibly accessible and shared so that the team would all know how their interactive services were working to help the patient live the best possible daily life. According to most of the service providers they had never before seen such a well-organized and documented health care system. If a new person became a provider, it was his/her job to read the daily notes to know what has been done, what is expected to be done, and how to report their results during their shift to help make the next caregivers services as productive as possible. This concept was an evolution of experience and learning from truly knowledgeable communicable managers, colleagues, and mentors during this experience and throughout my life. Because of the feedback from many healthcare professionals, I was inspired to write about it.

Now to introduce you to what I am referring to as the "Three Amigos of Many Hats." Three notebooks, in paper format, that ultimately contain every bit of information you will need as time passes and the caregiving journey follows its path. Let's begin to gather, compile and place the information that will help you through most any situation that may arise when you must step up to assist someone or be assisted.

The Purple Notebook – Daily Activities

This binder is for daily information and notes that will help answer health questions about daily living, health issues that are often forgotten by the time someone goes to the Physician or is needing medical care. The organizational information is designed to help the team that will gradually develop for caregiving. Also, a printed calendar will be a central information location so everyone on the team will know what is to happen and when or what has happened and why.

In case of emergency information is easily logged into the notebook. During a 911 call a common question asked by the dispatch person is, "what is the closest intersection to the address/location?" This is difficult enough to think about in an emergency situation when it is your own home but if it is someone else's address, it can be nearly impossible to know without using a GPS, which is a time-consuming task. The cross street and other quickly needed information can be written in this notebook along with who to contact in case of emergency (ICE) such as family or neighbors. Copies of healthcare surrogate, power of attorney, DNR, etc. can also be placed in this notebook for easy access at any time.

- Purple Notebook Examples of Information

- Quick Reference Information About US and Our Home

- Daily Calendar

- Medication List

Daily Caregiver Notes (all caregivers if multiple people) and service providers should use these daily notes for communication.

- In Case Of Emergency expanded information section, copies of POA, DNR, Health Directives.

- Copy of Power of Attorney

- List of Important Personal Information documents locator

The White Notebook – Health Information

This is an information guide to what most of us keep in our heads, in a filing cabinet, in a pile somewhere or on our phones. It contains important contact information of professionals who are in charge of our care and the chronological order of current care provided and over a lifetime. This may seem too simplistic, but when a person has had surgeries over a 20- or 50-year period, who else knows this information? Sometimes the list can be long or as with a Veteran, hospitalization could have been in a foreign country or at a VA Clinic in another State. A good example is people who have traveled for their jobs or led the life of career military, medical records can be stretched far and wide and trying to find out if someone had a gallbladder, or some other organ removed could be ancient history and who can remember all the details forty years later? A person could have pins and screws in their hand from a childhood accident or their tonsils out as a teen, where was the surgery done, when was the surgery done? The answers begin to fade no matter a person's age. We store so much information in our brain, sometimes the files are overfilled and accessing that information under the stress of examination becomes vague or even inaccessible. No one wants to believe they have some kind of memory failure! But it happens in times of stress or injury. Write this stuff down or have someone help you and do not worry about it again. It will be there on paper, in black and white, and easily accessible.

This book is something I wish I had had instead of bags of folders and boxes of records to sort through to find information. It was never easy and was a continual point of frustration until the organization began to materialize. It is my wish that this helps others to avoid the gauntlet of chaotic paperwork and information.

A healthcare provider is often hesitant to provide all medical records for someone. This takes extra time and office supplies to print someone's medical record history. But, if possible, it is helpful to have a summary or timeline for all office visits to include in the notebook. A patient must sign a request for medical records to be released and is worth the effort. The most recent records can be included in this notebook.

White Book Examples of information:

- Personal Health Information such as surgeries, injuries, chronic illnesses past and present.

- Healthcare professionals such as Physicians, Medical Facilities, Hospitals, Rehab Facilities, VA Clinics, Medical Equipment providers, past and present.

- Chronological order of healthcare summaries and physician visits for last two years. Older documents can be filed. A note should be made of where they are kept.

The Green Notebook – Confidential, Estate and Legal

This notebook may present the biggest challenge and once created should be kept in a secure location. The information it contains is mostly legal and financial. This can be one of the most important compilations of information secondary to personal health information. Copies of some of these original documents such as Power of Attorney, Healthcare Surrogate, DNR (Signed do not resuscitate) should be kept in the white notebook. If not, information about where to locate these documents needs to be in the white notebook. Original documents not stored in a person's home should be included on the Essentials List Locator with a description of what they are and where they can be found. There is an "Essentials List Locator" in Section 4 of Appendix Organizational Notebook Pages with blanks to fill in location of each item on the list.

A few examples of legal documents would be real estate documents for someone who owns rental properties. Properties would be listed and the location of the documents for the properties would be listed. All assets would be listed and the holder such as an Attorney, an Asset Manager, a safety deposit box, or relative, would be listed for each item. No more guess work for anyone at any time.

Why do this? To help facilitate the care of someone. Often people become very protective and private about their life's work, assets, and personal information. Ask any attorney or a family member who has gone through financing someone's care. If a person has assets to liquidate, this is a plus to help potentially keep them in their home with in-home services. If a person wants to move to a congregate living facility, knowing what assets are available to sell to finance a move and provide for long term care will be paramount. These facilities will require some of this information in order to qualify to move in. Some people have set up trusts. These come in a variety of flavors. Here are a few; revocable trust, irrevocable trust, Special Need Trust, Spendthrift Trust, Testamentary Trust, Generation Skipping Trust, Living Trust. Any of these may be called something different depending on the State in which it was created. The latter are called Family Trusts. As a caregiver it is not your job to know what these are, but knowing how to locate the Attorney or financial advisor is a must! They will help you through the labyrinth of issues if they arise.

As a caregiver, knowing that provisions have been made with a proper Power of Attorney and who holds that document will be one of the most important pieces of information. Having the proper legal documents when carrying out tasks such as paying bills or making decisions for someone else is necessary.

Also, important to remember, is that a Power of Attorney is only usable while someone is living. It is important to consult an Attorney to find out if someone's assets and liabilities are setup properly once he/she passes. In this notebook there is a detailed questionnaire that can be completed for "Final Arrangements."

Another reason to use this three-notebook organizational system is to help keep someone from taking advantage of a person needing care. Too often elderly are taken advantage of by someone who falsely makes them believe that they care. There have been documented situations when a deceptive person has influenced someone to change their will, change their power of attorney, or trusts. Making sure that all of the binders are used may not completely deter but will help to establish communication norms that dissuade someone who shows a desire to be the one and only person to be in control. Sharing information is important for the health and safety of the person needing care.

Here is another important reason to use these notebooks. An example of taking control, which has been shared by more than one person, is about family members who live in different states or parts of the world at the time a parent or family member needs care. Usually, one person is in charge. That person may have children who are supportive of the parent and decide they are also in charge of care. One person must be the "Captain of the Ship." Therefore written communication will save any caregiver from this scenario. So, the decision is made to not tell other family members what is going on with a loved one. This lack of communication may not be a coverup, but when outside family members are left in the dark theories arise and resentment can flair. The caregivers may feel the added communication required to keep others informed is more than they can handle. But and this is a big one, if these notebooks are used on a daily basis, a simple phone picture, scan of these pages and email or text with picture can ward off a potential family feud or added emotional disaster.

Green Book Examples of Information:

- Important Documents Locator List for easy reference.

- Attorney and Accountant Information – what service they provide.

- Power of Attorney – Original or where to find.

- Personal Financial Information - Originals or Location where to find originals.

- Estate Planning Documentation or Location where to find.

Takeaways:

- Refer to Chapter 11 "How To Organize Everyday Paperwork" Parts 1, 2, & 3 for guidance and instructions about how to assemble these binders. They may be purchased as a complete set also.
- An Attorney should always be considered and consulted when caring for someone else. Establish communication with the attorney with clear roles and responsibilities as the caregiver.

CHAPTER

6

Healthcare Management Gauntlet

Once you are in the labyrinth of healthcare.

Everyone's caregiving situation will be different. Being prepared as best as possible is what this book is about. Will all the answers be within these pages? No. Will you be the best prepared caregiver possible by reading this book and following its suggestions? Absolutely!

When thrown into a situation of four hospitals in three cities within three weeks I wished I had had this book to walk me through the gauntlet. It would have relieved me of the stress of trying to figure out what to do and how to find out information that would help. I could have avoided days ending with no progress made and succumbing to crying not knowing what to do next or to whom to turn.

But what about patient advocates and case managers?

Do not get me wrong, advocates and case managers are wonderful and helpful, they have big hearts and an extremely busy workload. The challenges with healthcare advocates and case managers are their limitations and inconsistency spanning across health and insurance institutions. These are not personal traits of an advocate, but their job limitations. Most every Hospital and insurance company has their own healthcare advocates. Without knowing this, as a caregiver we can end up communicating with a stream of people who have completely different interests regarding patient care and when called they regretfully say they cannot help. Why, you may ask? Because their help is limited to the care a patient receives in the facility that employs them. So be aware, each institution will have their own advocates who will help a caregiver/family member within the limits of the institution in which the patient is currently residing. Once no longer within the institutions care, an advocate can no longer provide guidance. This is just a fact and has nothing to do with good or bad care or the idea that no one cares.

Can I Hire a Medical Advocate?

There is also the option to pay for a medical advocate, this advocate can be hired. Be overly cautious when hiring someone as an advocate. Here are a few questions to get you going if considering hiring someone.

- What is your geographic location? Making sure the advocate is at least in the same town is helpful for family members who live out of town.

- How long have you been a medical advocate? Request references from other families who have used them and ask for permission to talk with those who gave references.

- How do you charge for your services? Hourly, weekly, monthly.

- Will charges be invoiced, and can the bill be paid by credit card?

- What are your working hours?

- In case of emergency, how do you respond?

- Have you handled similar situations to our needs?

- What do you consider a stressful situation?

- Are you bonded, insured and is your company technology HIPPA compliant?

- What are your credentials?

As of this publishing there may be some insurances that pay for an independent medical advocate service. No guarantee. Most Medicare and Medicaid insurances have an advocate or case manager that can help navigate the craziness of what is paid for and what is not. This includes services provided in healthcare institutions, at home or as an outpatient. This happens often when someone needs a service such as physical therapy. An insurance advocate/case manager will provide information and coordinate services ordered by a physician. Also, an insurance advocate can be helpful with scheduling home nurse visits for evaluations. This option is preferable to loading up a loved one who has mobility issues and trying to get them into a doctor's office.

Also, an insurance advocate knows what can be done through insurance, which is so important! If the situation arises that a patient would rather not receive care, this advocate can recommend a nurse to discuss other options such as Hospice. This takes the burden off of the patient and the family for this exceedingly difficult conversation. The advocate does not make the decision but knows the process to make sure a person's wishes can be fulfilled if he/she qualifies. Important, if an insurance provider is changed so is the advocate.

When someone can no longer manage their self-care and with no one from an institution who sees the big picture of coordinating a persons' care, a knowledgeable caregiver fortified with data is the best advocate for a friend or family member. No one can do it better in the short or long term!

Take Aways:

-   A caregiver is the leader of a team. The advocate/case manager is a member of the team but represents an institution unless privately hired.
-   Advocates/Case Managers scope of assistance is limited by their employer.
-   A team is comprised of many people to care for someone when he/she can no longer care for themselves and their daily living tasks. Congregate Living (Chapter 8) can offer a built-in team and advocate. At home a team must be assembled and the "How to Organize Everyday Paperwork" notebooks in Chapter 11 are an essential for easier management.

The Legal Gauntlet – Part 1 of 3

A practical guide to an impractical legal world.

DISCLOSURE/DISCLAIMER: The author nor anyone associated with this writing or publication is or claims to be an attorney or is providing legal advice. The information within this writing is strictly an opinion of definitions based on experiences and/or experiences from others shared with the author. No part represents specific people or situations and should not be construed as sharing personal information or outside the laws of any State or Central Government. Any commonalities felt are strictly because we are all touched by the human experience of caregiving at some point in our lives. The Gauntlet of Caregiving has no affiliation with any organizations mentioned and is not responsible for the content of their information materials or websites.

"I am just trying to help take care of my loved one!"

In the world of legalese and healthcare protectiveness, the system that has been set up to protect individual rights often interjects a wall between a person needing care and the caregiver. "The Legal Gauntlet" presents many challenges to a Caregiver whether caring for a relative or non-relative.

My Mother did everything right. Caregiving for her I had no issues working through this gauntlet. But sadly, it was more challenging helping others with whom I was personally involved. It became apparent that this gauntlet is one of the harshest and most challenging to maneuver through if everyone involved is not properly prepared for it.

More often than not we are unaware that normal purchases such as a home, vehicle, or anything that has a title showing the legal owners can escalate into a legal menace or battle when tragedy strikes. My Son experienced this at an early age. When my daughter-in-law had her second stroke from an aneurism that resulted in her being in a coma for a period of time. It was necessary to reduce expenses and bring her home for care. In order to sell the vehicle they owned together and buy a handi-van, this vehicle had to be sold. The car title was in both names as his "and" hers. It took a court appearance and judgement to sell the vehicle. Meanwhile payments had to be made or the risk of losing the vehicle and the potential for financial insolvency loomed. Sounds absurd. Well, this is a good example of the legal system that protects people. Knowing the outcome of an "if this, then" equation, is why it is important to consult an Attorney. I would not have believed this before, but it is true. Our life decisions must consider outcomes from a legal contractual perspective even when our world feels as though it is falling apart around us.

Regarding real property that has a legal title, the consequences of one party being incapacitated at some point must be considered. It reeks of distrust not only between partners or family members, but there are situations when titled assets must be disposed of in order to care for a loved one. The Durable Power of Attorney is the document that tells the legal community and financial institutions who can sell assets. It also can allow the Caregiver as "Agent" to handle bank accounts and other financial accounts for someone else while they are alive and incapable of performing these duties.

Having spent twenty plus years in real estate there have been many situations that have arisen regarding trusts. Trusts are meant to protect assets, designate beneficiaries, and allow for financial support for the next stage of life, healthcare, or perpetuity issues. The stories heard have been sad and sometimes tragic when family members do not understand how many different types of trusts are available. It is important to do homework here and once completed revisit what has been done at least every two to five years and update if needed. Become familiar with how many types of trusts are available for fulfilling specific situations. Talk to an attorney who knows trusts and have them explain pros and cons.

Then there is the healthcare realm where decisions must be made also. Why would a loved one not want you, the caregiver, to make medical decisions for him/her? Why would that be left up to those who work under the Hippocratic oath? What the heck is that oath anyway? Well, the healthcare workers are sworn to uphold ethical standards. But often are limited by financial parameters set by insurance providers, ergo the need for law to define patient rights. At least that is the way it appears to be set up. Attorneys have written the needed documents to help patients allow designated caregivers to have a say in someone else's treatment process. Take time to learn about the healthcare surrogate and healthcare directives.

The Birth of HIPAA

The Health Insurance Portability and Accountability Act generally is shortened to the acronym HIPAA. It is the fiercest opponent in the Legal Gauntlet of Caregiving.

How to tame it and make it your friend rather than your most vicious adversary?

Look to Chapter 11 "How To Organize Everyday Paperwork" forms section for the "Important Personal Information" list. Compiling this information includes legal documents such as a Living Will, Healthcare Directive, Healthcare Power of Attorney, Durable Power of Attorney, Estate Planning, or information on contacts of a third party who may hold these documents. Having these documents is paramount.

I received a call on an ordinary day at the office. It was my daughter-in-law. All she said was "I need a living will." I began asking questions to no response. She repeated what she needed and said she was in the hospital. At that time, my son was on a Military deployment preparation assignment. I asked to speak to the nurse and was filled in on the situation. I compiled the forms needed, prepared them to send where instructed, then I received a call from my son. "Mom, can you go to my house and take care of the girls until I can get back home?" Well duh, I said to myself, the lightbulb going off, realizing he was gone, and my grandchildren were by themselves with a friend in another state. I then answered "Of course, whatever you need…" This was my daughter-in-law's first stroke. Little did we know that her complete recovery was destined to be compromised again in a few years causing permanent disabilities. If we had only had this book.

For our family, this was a challenging time. But as a Military Family, it seemed rather natural to circle around the ones in need and take care of them while my son continued to serve in the Army. I must say, the Military are incredibly supportive of their men, women, and families of active-duty personnel. My daughter-in-law had been active with other Military wives where they were stationed. It was such an uplifting experience for me to be present when there was a call from the Army Chief of Staff, General Dempsey, to congratulate my daughter-in-law on being selected as an "Army Spouse of the Year."

The Bottom Line usually needs a signature.

No age is immune to the potential of needing help from a Caregiver. I have no statistics for this statement, but adult children more often become caregivers for aging parents than other types of caregiving. What has become known through conversations and firsthand experiences is that age nor circumstance will create any variables when entering the "Legal Gauntlet." Age does not provide forgiveness for legal fop-as, socio economic status, lack of experience, or emotional trauma. You, as a Caregiver, and whomever wishes for your help, must prepare to have signatures on legal documents before they are needed. Not every State requires a Notary but check in Chapter 14 Resources for a link to review a list for your state specific requirements for legal document notarization.

There is an organization called There is an organization called 'Aging with Dignity. whos program 'Five Wishes' provides guidance regarding healthcare directives. It is a good place to begin. You may be able to pick up a free copy at any doctor's office or go online to their website and purchase a copy of the booklet titled "Five Wishes." A digital version is also available for purchase. The link is included in Chapter 14 Resources.

My wish is that you proceed with confidence holding your "Organizational Notebook" securely in tow. Be confident as a caregiver, you will be equipped to do the best possible for your friend or family member.

Takeaways:

- Any age can be affected by The Legal Gauntlet.
- HIPAA is not a caregivers' friend but can be tamed!
- Every State in America has different laws for acceptable legal documents, due diligence is required.

Chapter 14 Resources has links for 'Aging with Dignity' program 'Five Wishes' and Government website references.
How to Organize Everyday Paperwork Chapter 11.
How to Organize Everyday Paperwork downloads Chapter 13.

The Legal Gauntlet – Part 2 of 3
Healthcare Directive Documents Dissected

NOTE: Healthcare Instructional Documents are Legal Documents

Wanting to help someone is admirable. But often trying to talk to anyone about the importance of preparing these documents is like telling a chef how to cook. It can be considered many things, more often intrusive instead of helpful. Therefore, if you are hesitant to discuss what needs to be done but want to be helpful, print out the "Important Personal Information" list and give it to someone you care about.

How to approach the subject: Legal forms change, new information is required, so all documents should be reviewed every 2-5 years, this is not only good practice, but provides an excuse to talk about the subject when sharing the list of Important Personal Information with someone. You could also purchase a copy of this book and give it to someone you care about, so the ideas do not come from you alone. The goal is to help as many people as possible to be prepared for the future.

Advance Directive

This term is very confusing, and it took some time and research to realize that it is a general term for any or all of the following healthcare documents. It is a folder word that is used to ask if you have them. These documents are a part of what an Elder Law Attorney can prepare. Also, there are non-profits who can give guidance, "Five Wishes" is referenced in this section below.

Health Care Surrogate, Healthcare Proxy Designation

These documents are called different names in different states. It allows a specific person (Agent) to make healthcare decisions if someone cannot. Each State has different laws and requirements, so make sure the proper terminology and forms are used for the state where the patient has his/her domicile or primary residence.

NOTE: HIPAA is a Federal Law, so all States must comply. There is a summary link to the requirements of HIPAA in Chapter 14 Resources.

Medical or Healthcare Power of Attorney

Some states require this instead of or in conjunction with a Health Care Surrogate or Healthcare Proxy Designation document.

Living Will or Healthcare Directive

This is a document stating the wishes of the patient when certain healthcare situations arise such as life support or prolonging medical treatments. Sometimes the information on this document is an opposing view of the caregiver. Consult with an Attorney when it comes to these kinds of decisions. It is difficult to discuss the "what if" scenarios, but when the time comes knowing that a loved one has chosen what he/she wants, and those wishes will be honored is important. (See DNR)

Healthcare Proxy

Allows a person to be appointed such as a Guardian, to make medical decisions when the patient cannot or will not. An example would be once someone accepts Hospice, a professional nurse or case manager is usually appointed to this position on the wishes of the patient or family. Or if a person is in a coma, unable to speak, write, etc.

If a situation arises and a person who needs care refuses to cooperate and it could be life threatening, there are resources to help. This can be considered self-neglect. It is a difficult situation for a caregiver, especially without documents designating authority. Help can be sought out through adult protective services in the state where the person resides. Having documentation of the situations leading up to the time of asking for help is especially important. This will provide the agency with tangible evidence to evaluate their first steps to help the person in need.

DNR: Do Not Resuscitate

In the world of healthcare, this document is considered a Healthcare Directive. An Attorney's advice should be considered regarding required duties and options as a Caregiver and Healthcare Surrogate. It is common practice for healthcare professionals to ask if someone of retirement age has a formal DNR. In many fifty-five and older age restricted communities it is common to see DNR notices on refrigerators. These documents are usually required to be signed by a physician and the person. If you have read previous chapters, one of my "Mom" moments mentions an experience with choosing to allow the use of an AED or defibrillator even though there was a DNR posted in the home.

Since DNR's is a part of a healthcare plan, a physician is usually the one to discuss it with a patient and sign the documents. Once someone choses Hospice Care a DNR will most likely be initiated as part of the continuing care plan. Depending on the State, using an Attorney to decipher the documents and assure that the documents are created and valid for the situation and location where it will be used, is a good practice. Also an Attorney can help with what happens if/when a DNR is put into use.

To sum it up

If you are a do-it-yourself kind of person who is comfortable using a generic legal form provider, be sure that the documents meet the State requirements of the resident to whom you are giving care resides. If you move the person from one state to another, make sure all documents are updated to meet legal requirements where the final residency is located. Otherwise, having any of these documents that cannot be honored is a moot point and the gauntlet wins!

As mentioned previously, after much research I found FiveWishes.org. This non-profit organization has all of the Healthcare Directive documents available for any state and offers a search capability. The documents are low cost and available in either paper copy or digital format. You can often receive a paper copy of "Five Wishes" pamphlet at no cost by asking for it from most any physician's office or healthcare facility. There is a sample of the front/back of this pamphlet included with the forms package.

The Legal Gauntlet – Part 3 of 3
What to talk about and who to talk to about it.

The nitty gritty!

This entire section has touched our family in one way or another. Always default to an Attorney for your personal needs. The most important information you can provide is the entire thought-out plan with any contingencies if situations change. Put all personal feelings aside and let the person who is choosing what to do go forward with your blessing.

As my husband and I traveled across the USA one summer in 2017 on our way to take his 88-year-old mother to see the Stampede in Calgary Canada, I received a call. My son was at the hospital with his wife. She had had another stroke from a brain aneurism that had been diagnosed and repaired seven years prior. It was a dire situation and fast forward she survived through many months of hospital and rehab facility submissions. As a result, she was physically disabled. Her husband, my son, became a 24/7 caregiver at age 38. At this young age few are prepared for the "Legal Gauntlet" that can potentially bankrupt and emotionally impact a family. All I can say is he is an amazing person and I have been blessed to learn so much from him as we all entered this crazy legal vortex!

Any age can be affected by The Legal Gauntlet. It is better to have written communication of a person's wishes than to leave the decisions to the healthcare and legal systems or

Government. Saying this is not to insinuate they are bad institutions, just that a person's decisions and wishes are the most important concern when he/she is not able to speak for themselves.

When asked to be an Agent for someone, accompany that person to their Attorney's office. Ask specific questions regarding the Power of Attorney duties and acceptable situations for implementation.

REMEMBER: An attorney represents their client who is the originator of the legal document. As the attorney, he/she does not represent you as the Agent.

Attorney Specialties Dissected

It is important to understand the differences in the abilities of Attorney's in the field of legal consultation and document preparation. Often people refer to an Attorney as their all-encompassing legal consultant when in reality not all attorney's practice all types of law.

Here is a list of different types of Attorneys that may be consulted when it concerns a person's welfare, assets, estate, and business. The list goes on with many specialties. For the purposes of caregiving, the following would be the primary specialists to address legal issues with someone who is aging or disabled.

Elder Care Lawyer
Bankruptcy Lawyer
Estate Planning Lawyer
Business Lawyer (Corporate Lawyer)
Family Lawyer
Real Estate Lawyer
Tax Lawyer

When it comes to pre-planning, choosing an Attorney is a personal choice. In small towns there may be a limited number of specialists available. Believe it or not, there are still small towns in America! If you are a caregiver moving to take care of a loved one, do not expect to have the same resources someplace else. Some Attorney offices have specialty lawyers of every kind, usually the offices with many names listed. Some are a one-person-band offering multiple services. The single Attorney office usually specializes and refers to others for areas of expertise. If they do not, proceed with caution!

Estate Attorney vs Elder Attorney

An Estate Attorney plans what will happen to a person's assets after death.

An Elder Attorney, or often listed as Elder Care Attorney, helps the elderly population and others to plan for life-changing events in their health. This specialist can help with VA benefits, Medicaid, and other qualified health care options. Having an Elder Care Attorney in situations such as caring for a friend, a family member when multiple family members are involved, or to learn what options can be initiated for care when needed can be greatly beneficial to the person needing care. It is a good option to relieve family members from the stress of making health care decisions and provisions.

POA Legal Documents Dissected

Power of Attorney Variants.

I mention variants because a power of attorney can be specific in what it allows someone to do for someone else. From experience, it is important to know ahead of time exactly what is expected and accepted by the entity that will be needing the document i.e.: banks, real estate brokerages, courts, healthcare facilities. Also, there are different types of documents and knowing the purpose and difference is important.

Example: Real estate transactions need to be specific, clearly stating the duties to be performed by the "Agent." Agent is what the designated substitute is named. This is why an Attorney should be consulted. Giving complete control to sign anything and everything including the sale of a home and/or properties, a vehicle, boat, etc. could be legally dangerous and financially devastating. There are too many terrible stories about an elderly person ending up without anything and destitute because of someone they entrusted to do the right thing! Never allow someone else to have their attorney create legal documents that involve you and your assets. Always speak directly with an attorney as the client!

As a caregiver it is important to always default to involving the person until they can no longer participate. Yes, you have Power of Attorney, but it should be used only with permission from the person who has assigned it to you. The ability to participate is not a decision for the caregiver to make! Always have a witness or consult with the Attorney who created the document prior to implementing it. Even on a case-by-case basis, never assume responsibility for a monetary transaction of any kind! Why? It is a CYA. Cover your assets! Know that there may be disgruntled people in line to inherit that 1950's rust bucket car or that old, cracked vase that was actually a Ming vahz. Helping could put your personal assets at risk to settle an estate. You may never know who is in a person's will. From experience, to say the least it can be surprising!

Durable Power of Attorney vs Regular Power of Attorney

These two documents are distinctly different. Having encountered both, it is a challenge to say which is most important. It is up to the individual and their comfort level.

The Durable Power of Attorney can be used while the person is capable of participating or if he/she becomes disabled, incompetent, or incapacitated. This document relies on the complete trust of the individual who is the designated Agent.

The General Power of Attorney is only usable by the Agent while the designator is able to participate. This is often used to assign an Agent with designated duties to operate in their absence.

Example: A married couple are buying a home. One has to leave town and only one is available to close on the property. This type of document can be used to provide legal authority for the one person to sign closing documents in the absentee's stead. These days with digital document signing and overnight shipping capabilities often this is not used any more. Caution, this document must be written correctly in order to be honored by all parties involved including but not limited to State law, financial institution requirements, and Federal law. It is best to consult an Attorney and provide every step that is planned so the document can be prepared correctly. Otherwise, it will be useless.

NOTE: Some States may allow for a General Power of Attorney with a Durable Power of Attorney add on. Consult a local Attorney in the State where the document will be used.

Also Note: If the issuer has properties in multiple States to be handled by a designated Agent, there should be a Power of Attorney specifically for each State where the properties are located.

Is the Power of Attorney everlasting? So often people assume the Power of Attorney is a forever document. It is not. It is only meant to help handle the legal and financial affairs for someone else during their life.

A Power of Attorney becomes void after Death

Many, including myself, innocently with good intentions make promises about continuing to help someone after they are gone. But once a person has passed, the final "Will and Testament" takes precedence over all else. In order to keep this simple, if you offer to take care of a person's belongings or continue to feed their cat by accessing the property after that person has passed you could be breaking the law. Yes, this is true.

When a person has passed, and a "Will" takes over what is to happen to a person's assets, a caregiver must have instructions on how to proceed or desist. Yes, this would include taking care of the beloved cat or other pets. Good intentions can be hindered by the lack of written communication about so many things. Helping someone else or yourself to be prepared is hopefully why you are here. Have intentions in writing and notarized!

As a Realtor® I have worked with many people who have been in a situation with the need to sell a parents' home in order for them to move on to the next level of care in a facility. Family members have come to me with many kinds of permissive documents that allow them to sell someone else's real property. Many times, there is confusion regarding those rights. Often, the property owner has had to sign for an updated Power of Attorney which must be created by the original Attorney. Homes in certain types of Trusts can go on for generations. These documents have caused some remarkably interesting struggles in the "Legal Gauntlet." In more than one situation over a half-century had passed, the Attorney who wrote the Trust had passed and the Attorney who held the Trust had to make some major adjustments because of the language written within the trust no longer complied with changes in the Laws governing Trusts. Luckily in several situations over the years the Trustee was still alive to agree and assign a new Trustee. Sadly, in one situation, the trustee passed not long after this was completed. It worked out for the heirs and plans could move forward.

When you have all of the legal documents in order, catalog them in your "Organizational Paperwork Notebook" legal folder. Only keep a copy of the Power of Attorney (not an original) in the Purple daily activities and White health information folder. Often this is enough to give permission to speak on someone else's behalf. The Green "Confidential Estate and Legal" notebook is where Certified or stamped copies should be kept unless they are held by an Attorney. The "Locator List of Essential Information" can reference documents held elsewhere. This notebook is best kept in a safe place and can be provided to whomever requires it upon request. Original documents are usually required for financial institutions such as banks, closing agents for real estate transactions, and many other situations. If these documents are not available to you, make sure to note where each document is being held. If held at an Attorney's office, set up a preliminary appointment to establish how to obtain copies of them when needed. Once completed, as a Caregiver, you will be prepared for pretty much anything legally required.

The Locator List of Essential Information is a certainty for locating documents of every kind. It should be revisited at least annually to make sure it is up to date.

Here are a few questions to ask about being an Agent as a caregiver. These questions will provide an opportunity for the Attorney to inform not only you, but their represented client as well. Stating the answers in front of the person who will be taken care of will help them to know and understand the implications of the power of the document and the responsibilities they are asking of the caregiver.

When is the best time to use or implement the use of a Power of Attorney?

In what ways can this Power of Attorney be used?

What is the Agent's obligation to use the document?

Can the Agent be changed at any time, if changed, how will Agent/caregiver be notified?

If applicable, how does this affect a Trust? In other words, can the POA change a Trustee? This is important for the person creating the document to understand. Example: Spouses create a trust naming each other as trustees. One of them passes before the other. The remaining person becomes aged or incapacitated. Who then can change a trustee if the current trustee is not able to do so?

If the person passes away, are the bank accounts "In Trust For" a beneficiary so that bills can continue to be paid since the Power of Attorney is no longer useful.

Do it yourselfers, proceed with caution! Make sure to have witnesses and a Notary to notarize documents. Doing it yourself in this way is not recommended but it is legal. There are legal forms available online for a fee.

Regarding banking accounts with (POD) payable-on-death or (TOD) transfer-on-death naming a beneficiary. This is a situation I would never have thought about if I had not encountered the repercussions of bank accounts becoming non-accessible upon death.

IMPORTANT NOTE: When becoming someone's caregiver, talk to the attorney or the bank about what happens to the account upon death. Like so many others in caregiving, this is not a comfortable question to ask. Just know when a bank account has no assigned beneficiary, upon death the account can be frozen until probate is completed. What this means is that a home could sit without utilities, without insurance, and all too often can go into foreclosure during the time of probate. I have personally seen properties sit for years, become totally abandoned and then sold off by financial institutions for pennies on the dollar or by municipalities for back taxes. Even investment properties could be at risk. Tenants cannot pay rent or stop paying rent, the estate loses money, taxes and insurances are not paid. Ask an attorney how single-member LLCs without a beneficiary are handled. A real nightmare! Do not let this happen to your loved ones' assets they worked so hard to accumulate. If an attorney or an individual is assigned to handle an estate, they will not be able to access funds either without an assigned beneficiary either.

Takeaways:

- Compile all documents listed in the "Locator List of Essential Information" and include them in the designated "Organizational Paperwork" folders for easy access.
- Power of Attorney is a document that can be all encompassing or specific. Know what you want to do with it so it can be written correctly. This document is no longer usable after death.
- The Last Will & Testament and Executor come into play after death. Never promise to take care of a person's belongings after passing, you could be breaking the law.

The Gauntlet of Congregate Living

A guide to what is and what is not.

Congregate Living 101

Feeling beat up by why there is not one facility that offers all of what is needed to take care of someone? Welcome to the Gauntlet of Congregate Living.

If you have not experienced moving someone in and out of facilities because the services that were available did not meet what was needed, you are not alone. It is not the facility; it is the Healthcare industry and the Government protecting individuals from themselves that has limited how these facilities can provide care. This is just a fact, not a grievance. As you read on, it will become clear why more people are giving up careers to take care of someone at home. There were some good things that came out of the pandemic, remote working was one. More people are able to work and stay home to be caregivers when needed these days. Having said this does not mean it will be easy, there is a formula that works in the remote working environment that needs to be considered and every industry has its requirements.

What is congregate living? In short, this kind of living situation entails housing a person or family in a private room. This room can be the size of a bungalow, small condo/apartment, a hotel room, or a double occupancy hospital style room. A congregate living situation could be in a converted home also. These living accommodations are usually in a specific building or within a development that complies with State laws as a congregate living facility. What makes it congregate living is the management and amenities. A central food service is usually set up as a dining room with specific serving hours, activities rooms, social services, housekeeping, beauty salon, and a plethora of other added amenities/services.

So now that the congregate living option has been defined, why are there so many types of facilities? This is where the Gauntlet challenge arises. If someone you care for needs 24/7 care, Assisted Living may not be the best choice. The term "assisted" is very well defined by governance, but not as most of us assume. Much stress can be caused by the need for help and the idea that what we thought would be a solution ends up being an extremely expensive and unhelpful mistake. Even if someone has stated that he/she would move into a facility when needing a certain level of care, it does not mean it is the best option for future care. Often by the time someone decides to move they do not qualify for independent or assisted living.

Congregate Living Dissected

In the Resources page there is a list of acronyms for congregate living facility types you can review. There are also website addresses if you are interested in reading more from the sources. It is important to understand what the acronyms mean when you are engaged in conversations with a facility or a placement agency. It will be helpful to ask good questions to receive specific answers. This process will eliminate any assumed conclusions about what services will be provided, are included or when there will be a cost for additional services. Also, it is important to know that other than Age-restricted communities, any community that offers services to someone will have health status requirements. So be prepared with your health information and financial paperwork, power of attorney, health care surrogate, living will and DNR or healthcare power of attorney paperwork! Refer to the "Data Dump Gauntlet" (Chapter 5) and "How to organize everyday paperwork" (Chapter 11) sections for guidance.

Placement agencies are everywhere. These agencies are not advocates for someone's care. They are referral agencies for local facilities and are compensated for their referrals. The service can save time researching, but also depending on the location in the United States, not all facilities or options may be forthcoming because the agency does not receive compensation. Just being candid here, these agencies do not work for free. It is important to have all the facts when considering help for contracting with a residential community. This information is to be used as awareness not negativity, nor endorsement or non-indorsement.

Age-Restricted Communities

Age-restricted communities usually require at least one resident to be of a certain age. Always check the rules and regulations. Ask if there is a percentage of non-fifty-five-year-old residents if a future caregiver does not meet the age requirement. This happens frequently; an adult child becomes a caregiver and needs to move in with Mom and Dad to take care of them, but the homeowners association will not allow it because of his/her age. This scenario can cause emotional, physical and financial burden on families. For this reason alone it is very important to check age requirements prior to buying in a community to see if there is a possibility of needing care by someone under the specified age allowed.

Often these communities are not congregate living facilities. Instead, these communities offer independent living, usually in a home style setting which are houses of many sizes, modular style homes or condominiums. These differ from an Independent Living Community because there are no professional services provided. It is strictly an age-restricted dwelling which means no one under a certain age is allowed to live there full time unless they are a significant other or spouse and one of them meets the age requirements. Some communities have percentages of allowable underage residents.

Independent Living Communities

Independent Living communities or facilities come in all different configurations these days. The common thread is what services are offered to their residents. There are veritable menus of service options, and it can be mind boggling to say the least. Here are a few common communities found in most areas of the United States.

Progressive Care Buy in Options:

These facilities are usually built like a micro development and have boundaries with beautiful gardens, country club style amenities and may offer different levels of independent living. A large home, villa or luxury condominium can be an option. The buy in cost reflects the options selected and basically once a person has "bought in" they are guaranteed to receive whatever level of living care needed for the duration of their ability to afford this choice, at a locked in price.

This option comes with a hefty price tag but knowing that financial planning has taken the costs into account, it can provide a feeling of freedom and independence.

Progressive care would include moving within the community from an independent to assisted, then to assisted with nursing options and/or nursing home or long-term care if needed. A wonderful option for those who have carefully planned their financial future.

Progressive Care Rent Options:

This kind of community, sometimes called continuing care, is extremely popular. It often has an option for residents to move on to the next level of care within the facility because of their residency without escalated costs. There are more of these types of facilities available now than ever before because a large number of the population just need to control the cost of living. This kind of facility is usually a condo/apartment style building on a large property with easy access using elevators and paved sidewalks. They will have a full kitchen, but residents are provided with a main meal and snack each day. A central dining room provides the meal for the day and other optional foods can be ordered from a limited menu. Every building is easily accessible, and amenities are in a central location like a country club. There are also many options for additional services such as being driven to appointments in the facility provided car, free maintenance for the dwelling, food delivery, and more.

Independent Living only:

Independent living is a catch phrase for many kinds of living options that provide everything except individual care. If a person cannot take care of themselves such as personal hygiene, feeding and clothing themselves, he/she cannot qualify to be independent. Every person applying to reside in this type of community will be evaluated by a healthcare professional to make sure health requirements for independence are met. Basically, you have to be completely independent to qualify. Often people are, well, independent and do not look at this type of facility until it is too late to qualify because they need more help to accomplish daily tasks. This is great for people who like the fee added options when needed or want additional services such as having laundry done, main meals provided, housekeeping, concierge services for drivers to appointments, etc. Or for those who like social activities right where they live!

Assisted Living:

This type of living situation is not really what it says. But it does provide the services that are helpful when the next level of care is needed. Assisted living is similar to independent living in that there are strict health qualifications. Usually if a person needs support for ambulatory issues, medication dispensing, non-optional laundry, housekeeping which includes changing sheets and linens, and a menu of other helpful services, this is the place! Every additional service other than meals and basic housekeeping are usually an upcharge. When making a visit to an assisted living facility, you will see people in wheelchairs, using walkers, and in all stages of needing care. Yet they are all moving around, attending activities and not bed bound. This is important to remember. To live here a person must be as independent as possible considering their health situation. Anyone applying to live here must be evaluated by a healthcare professional to meet the facility requirements.

Nursing Home/Rehab Living:

Nursing Homes often are where people do not want to go. Many have become Rehab facilities for short term patients. Insurance companies often set a maximum number of days for a stay in this type of facility. Nursing homes are long-term facilities. Unless a person has long-term healthcare insurance a nursing home cannot be a long-term option. Here lies the confusion. Yes, anyone can stay long-term in a Nursing Home, but the cost is astronomical, or they must qualify for financial assistance. For this reason, the healthcare industry continues to reinvent itself to create a solution for the continuing need for the next level of care.

Regarding someone who is not a senior. Nursing Home/Rehab centers are not age specific; all of the other living options listed are. There are State/County congregate living options for all ages which includes adults with disabilities and are available through Medicaid social services. This is another subject entirely and an important one to be addressed later, on its own.

Home Away From Home:

This type of congregate living is usually in a neighborhood setting which is a home that has been converted into a small facility. Often the owner has decided to become a caregiver full-time and lives on premises with hired assistants that cover a 24/7 time period for the residents. In some parts of the country there may be corporate owned homes like this. These kinds of living opportunities are often much more like a home environment because there are a limited number of rooms available and a more intimate one-on-one caregiving service. The cost is surprisingly very reasonable compared to larger corporate facilities depending on the location and availability. From research the turnover is exceptionally low so often there is a waiting list. Be careful when previewing these kinds of homes. Make sure their credentials are available or references can be provided.

Stay at Home:

Believe it or not, this is an option! Since the pandemic of 2020, the government and the private sector have all worked to provide a solution to keep someone at home when in need of care. Of course, there are times when this is not an option or the person needing care has chosen one of the above-mentioned living situations and moved forward. For those who would prefer to stay home, this book has been written for this kind of caregiving. Sometimes long-term care is needed but not a viable financial option. What to do?

Stay at home with someone.

Hire an Agency caregiver.

Use State/County/City Senior Services

Signup for Medicaid and use their services.

Signup for Medicaid and check to see if compensation is available to be paid as a caregiver at home. Depending on the Government at both federal and state levels, a spouse may or may not be eligible for compensation.

Use Veteran or Spouse Aid & Attendance benefits

Every Government based program that covers the cost of Caregiving has a list of requirements to qualify for using the services. Refer to the Appendix for a list of Medicaid offices by State.

Every State establishes the financial income criteria to qualify for Medicaid. Go to the Medicaid website for your State to read the income and assets maximum. If a person cannot qualify for Medicaid due to income, contact a County or Municipality Council on Aging to ask about services. Often a person cannot have more than $120,000 in assets to qualify for non-Medicaid services. Once a person qualifies for Medicaid, local services will be discontinued. No double dipping or trying to hide assets. These services will review financial statements for the last five years (which could change at any time) to make sure assets and monies have not been moved. They cannot be hidden, be honest and be prepared!

At this time, for Medicaid, liquid assets must not exceed $2,000 in cash value. That means no more than $2,000 in a bank account at any given time, no car valued more than $2,000 in their name even if it has a loan. Also, the requirements change so keep up to date.

To qualify for Medicaid a person must require the level of care provided in a nursing home facility. The interviewer will go down a list which usually includes the need for help with feeding, clothing, bathing, general hygiene, walking/standing/ambulatory issues requiring walkers/wheelchair/lifts. If a person is bedridden, it is important to fully disclose this. Some agencies will not provide caregivers due to the risk of injury when lifting a patient. These are some generally acceptable issues and not a complete list.

Each State has it own way of calculating Medicaid income requirements. This means ANY income other than social security may go to offset expenses first. The answer to your question is NO. Medicaid will not allow a caregiver or family member to take income to maintain a loved one's home expenses when receiving services from Medicaid. Consult an Attorney to set up an estate plan ahead to take care of this potential issue.

Medicaid will review assets to prevent an applicant from giving away assets to qualify. Each State is different. Use the list of links in "Resources" (Chapter 14) to familiarize yourself with qualifications. Here are a few other options, be prepared to pay for some services:

Elder Law Attorney.
Geriatric Care Manager.
Eldercare Financial Planner.
Public benefits counselor/case manager.
State health insurance programs.
Commission based Medicaid planner.
Insurance agents.
Long term care ombudsman.
Self-planners.

Takeaways:

- Estate and financial planning are the best ways to avoid the financial burdens of long-term care.
- Familiarize yourself with the different types of services and facilities available.
- Evaluate cost of staying at home vs cost of a facility and paid services
- If you are a family member or friend, make sure you have legal documents in place to make decisions for someone. Knowing what you are doing means reading, asking questions, and doing research or you could end up financially responsible.

The Respite Gauntlet

Getting to know what you need

Respite care is defined as providing short term relief for a caregiver who is engaged in taking care of a sick, disabled, or elderly person.

I have personally experienced the help of an outside source for respite. Whether a person is a caregiver for a week, a month, a year or indefinite, respite is one of the most important experiences for a Caregiver.

As stated in the introduction to "The Gauntlet of Caregiving," a Caregiver will, out of necessity, more often than not, consider their needs or time for themselves, as not important or believe there is no time for consideration of what he/she needs. The daily job of a caregiver is not 9-5, 7-3, 11-7. The job becomes a lifestyle and along with "The Gauntlet of Merging Lifestyles," there is the need to take care of the Caregiver.

According to Aging Care "30% of Caregivers die before the people they care for do." Other sources quote much higher incidences of this phenomenon. Why? There are many reasons, but the most common thread is the lack of self-care.

A Mom Taught Me Moment: She knew me so well and having a tendency of being a caregiver to anyone who needed help, she would often tell me this when I became careless with taking care of my own needs.

"If you don't look after yourself, what good will you be to anyone else."

This section is written to help you, the Caregiver, be aware that taking care of another's needs is all consuming if allowed to be. If you are fortunate enough to have a large family and they are willing or able to help with the loved one who needs care, you are blessed. The story that seems most common is one family member, for whatever reason, is the only individual one out of many that becomes the Caregiver. So, for lack of statistics on this subject, the assumption here will be that it does not matter how many people are in a family, it could be an only child or a dozen siblings, more than likely there will be one primary Caregiver.

Recently a friend shared with me that he has been traveling once a month to help take care of his parents who live out of State, or in his case back home. With Siblings local to the parents, all have been taking turns. This is not the most common of situations and this family is truly blessed. Wouldn't it be wonderful if we all could have this kind of corroborative help for Respite Care? Yes, and you too can have a team.

A Team Effort

There are many people who have been caregivers and touched my life in ways that have inspired me to write about this important topic. One person in particular has spent a large portion of her life taking care of others. She cared for her father-in-law by bringing him into her home. Then her mother by bringing her into her home and she cared for her husband for years, fifteen of them while he was bedridden from Parkinson's disease. She endured the loss of two children during these years, initiated family celebrations such as birthdays, holidays, and other special occasions. All of these years of caregiving seem to come naturally to her. She did this while she raised children, worked, and did not question why, or how, as she would say, "you just get on with life and do what you need to do…"

There is one especially important trait that stands out about this amazing person. She knew when to take a break. She was never without responsibility or frivolous with her respite time but planned it carefully and sparingly through choice with the help of family so as not to burden them too much. She created a team of dependable people who would help when needed, it was just part of what needed to be done. As decades of Caregiving passed and she retired, she continued maintaining social circles with her club meetings, having a beloved gardening hobby, reading, collecting books, cooking, and encouraging family time with children, grandchildren, and great grandchildren. As of this writing she still lives independently with her sister now in her home and is in her mid-nineties. A true legend of inspiration. As of this writing she has, after ninety-five years, acknowledged the need to have a caregiver herself.

Taking a break to do a chore such as grocery shopping, having the car washed, going to lunch with a friend, getting outside to garden, art without interruption, or going to work and having a meal be ready when you get back, are important daily respite situations that are healthy and necessary.

So often Caregivers share that they are exhausted, mentally, and physically. Loneliness is one of the common threads that Caregivers have expressed. Yes, when one person is solely responsible for another and becomes socially isolated, it can be lonely. But as has been expressed in many ways, a person can be lonely in a crowd, or be happy alone. Surrounding yourself with others, taking a walk or reading a book can provide you with some off duty time and anything that helps you relax and refocus is a great way to take care of yourself. Add this personal time to the calendar!

Consistency is the Golden Key

To be consistent with scheduling respite care will meet several goals. First, consistent care of the loved one is paramount. If they are made aware that someone else will be visiting for a few hours so that you can go somewhere or do a chore, it will be expected even if he/she does not remember, put it on the calendar. Second, this "knowing" that you as the Caregiver will have 2-4 hours to yourself ahead of time gives you something to plan for and look forward to doing. It is easy to slip into what I term as the "Care-Funk." The professional name would be burn-out. What does this feel like? Extreme exhaustion, change in appetite, bad self-care such as lack of hygiene, avoiding doctor appointments, irritability or poor treatment when taking care of your loved one. There are other symptoms of this care-funk, but most importantly knowing it can happen to anyone at any time and planning for it can help to avoid major stress for you and your loved one.

How to avoid "Care-Funk." When you are faced with becoming a caregiver, begin finding out what outside help there is available for free or the cost of paid professionals. Here are some suggestions:

The VA, County, City, State, Medicaid, and Churches offer paid and volunteers for short term care. Having a friend or neighbor can be a short-term solution, but as "Merging Lifestyles" mentions, people are usually only good for short term visits, this situation is not a lasting solution. Once a Caregiver becomes dependent on a friend or neighbor the relationship runs a risk of disintegrating. It just happens. For long-term situations it is best if a professional or retired caregiver or nurse is hired. When filling out a calendar be sure to include days for "you" time. Usually, these times must be scheduled during the 9-5 workday when hiring outside help. If you have a family who can help often this option is best scheduled on weekends or evenings if they work. Sometimes if family members live out of town it may be a once a month, or once in a while situation. This is not something to depend on.

Chapter 14 Resources has information and links to information about home and community-based services for Medicare and Medicaid options.

If you contact a company to hire, the cost will be $27-$50 an hour. Often these companies like to have consistent days and hours for their professional Caregivers. The more hours you hire, the better the price. The best situation is to have the same caregiver help each time so that it creates a consistent environment for your loved one. When hiring a company or using Medicaid services this can be a challenge. Anyone who can be consistent is a treasure. Treat them as such.

For seniors there are resources such as "Senior Day Care" which provides a place where you can take your loved one for a few hours. Some are like child day care centers which allow for longer hours. But the cost varies and the exposure to others is sometimes not in keeping with the loved one's social comforts. It is worth trying it out.

Exploring Resources

Respite care for Caregivers is such an enormous subject that many research studies have been done encompassing many different caregiving scenarios. The actual industry has not caught up to the true need in my opinion. Having sought out resources for this kind of care, the end result is dependent upon the income of the patient/loved one. Medicaid for example may provide up to 40 hours of care. Usually, daytime. A state or County program may provide up to 20 hours of free care, also daytime and weekdays. For odd hours such as overnight or weekends a home health company would be the source of caregivers or healthcare professionals for an hourly fee. Any free services require qualifying financial information which has been mentioned before in Chapter 8 "The Gauntlet of Congregate Living". Another reason to have the "Data Dump" in Chapter 5 completed and updated as soon as possible.

The Veterans Administration has their own system of providing care for a Veteran or the surviving spouse of a Veteran. This system is called "Aid and Attendance." As with all things that are operated by the Government, it takes time to set up and be funded. There is an extensive application process with income and healthcare need qualifications. The funds received for Aid and Attendance must be paid to a Health Care Provider or private care giver. As a Veteran there are many more options for care available. At the time of this writing the benefit was up to $3,649 a month. This is not enough to hire someone full-time but can certainly provide plenty of respite care.

Since Covid-19 lockdown there have been some government programs that pay live-in caregivers instead of hiring someone to come in. As of this writing those programs are still available. Discuss this with the local Medicaid office to see if this is available where you live. The negative is that you cannot receive respite in this scenario from the city, County or State. You would need to rely on other resources in order to schedule the most important "you" time.

"A good laugh and a long sleep
are the two best cures for anything."
– Irish proverb

For more information regarding other options such as congregate living go to "The Gauntlet of Congregate Living" (Chapter 8) to read what it is and what it is not.

The A, B, C's of Self Care

Hah, you say! You raised children, have taken care of people or animals before. You know what it means to be responsible and take care of others. Well, that is all good experience, but… have you taken the best care possible of yourself?

When it comes to taking care of another individual it is paramount to take care of you. As mentioned in Chapter 4 "The Emotional Gauntlet of Merging Lifestyles," being a caregiver is not having someone adjust to your lifestyle. Sometimes the situation is out of your control. It is all about adjusting to their situation. What?

Being a caregiver can be a soul-searching event. The potential for burning out at some level is inevitable. It is human, especially if the idea that caregiving is extremely stressful in and of itself is not acknowledged. This is why Respite is a must.

Taking care of yourself also means communicating with people in your life, including professionals, that your life has changed. It has changed. Caregiving is a whole different level of giving and of caring.

One issue that arises is that no matter if a person is a friend or a family member, when you become a caregiver, the relationship changes. A good example of this change is to consider having an adult child move back home. Yes, he/she is still your child but not a child anymore. Instead, this child is an independent adult with life experiences lived without you being involved. To think that he/she is the same and should meet your expectations today can interfere with a new adult friendship/relationship. Respecting this change and difference can lead to a fulfilling experience. Trying to live together as you once did without acknowledging the change can cause stress for all. The same goes for someone being a caregiver.

Here are some steps to follow that can help you to help yourself.

Acknowledge the difference between you and the person you are caring for. Then find common ground. Refer to Chapter 4 for some questions that will help you get to know someone no matter how well you believe you know them.

Embrace the idea that they are the center of the caregiving universe. You are the ultimate giver!

Share your frustrations and caregiving issues with a professional. Whether you feel overwhelmed or not, this is a good thing. This does not mean you are weak, broken or not responsible!

Who do I speak with, you ask? Talk to your physician, a counselor or healthcare professionals who are coming in to provide respite. Be aware that friends and family may not be the best to air your personal issues with caregiving challenges you are facing taking care of someone whom they know and love. They will have many responses and soon may not respond. This does not mean stopping communicating with them about important issues regarding a person's care. Work to keep friends and family for happy respite visits with you to take care of yourself too.

Take care of your health, so that you can take care of someone else. Make a calendar for yourself. Block out time on a regular basis for fun activities as well as healthcare visits and exercise. Communicate with your caregiving team. Everyone will appreciate you taking time off to take care of yourself.

Read books on self-care. There are many.

Find a caregiving social group to connect with on social media. Be careful not to give personal information about you or the person you are caring for. Sometimes others will say things that may give you an "aha" moment. You never know when or where a bit of inspiration or a solution can happen.

Social groups such as church, clubs, or home neighborhood activities can be included on the calendar and provide something to look forward to outside of the caregiving world.

Plan daily small moments of self-care. Enjoy a cup or glass of your favorite beverage at a set time, if possible, each day. If a set time is missed, just delay, but do it! Treat yourself to something like a favorite snack or create a healthy option to look forward to. If a small piece of chocolate with a cup of coffee does the trick, go for it. This author tries to have a hot cuppa sweet milky tea at 2:00 each day (3:00 with daylight savings time). It is not always possible, so accomplishing the planned event is always a special and pleasant treat.

"Self-love seems so often unrequited."
-Anthony Powell, Author

Takeaways:

- You are important. Respite is self-care.
- The statistics vary. Research indicates 18%-30%+ Caregivers suffer ill health causing death before the person they take care of passes. Caregivers statistics of dementia or Alzheimer's patients are much higher.
- Use the resources as a guide to find help in your location. Ask questions of other friends and family who have been caregivers.
- Write respite time on the calendar IN INK so it is permanent!
- Go to "Resources" Chapter 14 for the HHS link and research home and community-based services in your area (HCBS) Home and Community Based Services.

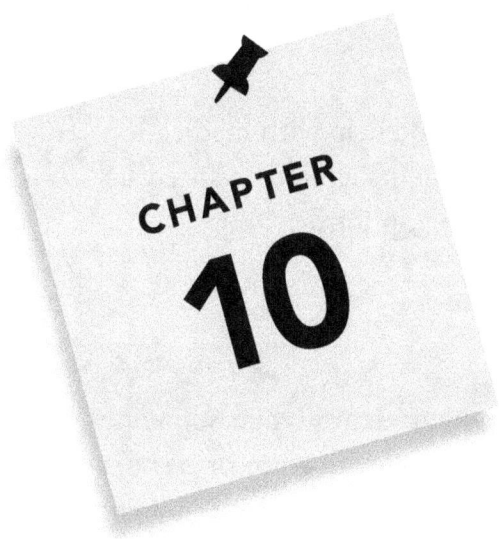

CHAPTER
10

Gauntlet of Medication Management

Danger… Danger… Danger!

When it comes to medication management, the repercussions can be extremely challenging. As an adult who has always managed his/her own life to be suddenly told that they are no longer capable of taking their own medication correctly is a huge deal. If not addressed, it can also be dangerous for the person's good health and safety.

Before going forward with any medication management options, all prescribing physicians should be consulted and agree with any changes!

There are many ways to handle medication management. But first it is important to approach the subject with a professional such as a physician or healthcare professional. Within the "Organizational Notebook" there is a blank list where medications can be listed. This list should correspond with the latest physician visit summary.

Once an updated list has been established an in-home inspection for extra or outdated medications should take place and any non-prescribed medications discarded*. This process is when disagreements can occur, and references should be used from the most recent physician visit to validate why you, the caregiver, are helping to fulfill the need to make sure old medications are disposed of and the proper medications are available for consumption.

In some cases, a nurse may be assigned to make home visits and help with medication management. This is a help and can often diffuse disagreements as well as speed up the transition process to an organized medication dispensing option.

Medication dispensing options

As with most things in life, medication dispensing is a conundrum when someone needs help to accomplish this task. Whether daily supportive medication or a short term needed regime, this is one of the most important daily actions for an individual. The current method of dispensing medications should be observed and the need for a change will depend on the individual's situation.

Here are a few examples of medication issues that should be addressed:

1. All prescriptions are stored in one place such as a drawer, cabinet in the bathroom, kitchen, or elsewhere.

Working with the person to look at the medications and make a list for reference will be a least invasive way to take stock in outdated medications (literally), old no longer needed, and relevant or current medications.

2. Observe how the person takes their medications. Does he/she have set times? Is a reminder device used such as a pill box? Is a timer set? Is it a list with a check off system already in place?

If any or all of the answers to these questions are no, to prevent accidents with an individual who may be starting with confusion regarding their medications, a complete review and discussion should ensue and using the "medication list" as a beginning works well.

3. There are many solutions to dispensing medications. Pill boxes for daily, weekly, and even monthly refillable options are available.

If an individual has a set routine with a specific pill storage/dispenser, it will be a huge challenge to help them create a new habit. So careful consideration needs to be given to the individuals capability to self-medicate.

4. Find a solution.

Today technology can be very helpful with electronic pill dispensers available that hold a months' worth of medication. The pros for this are many, including the ability to notify a third party automatically if medications are not taken. Then the receiver can call and remind the person to take the medication dispensed by the machine. The cons are few, but one is important which happened to the author. The machine cannot dispense half tablets. These machines are expensive and cost hundreds, the manufacturer allowed the machine to be returned because it was indeed a design flaw. So disappointing, this is a fantastic piece of technology!

How to prevent refills of no longer used medication:

Problem: Many prescriptions are automatically refilled. Why? Because many pharmacies will continue to refill a prescription automatically until refills need a doctor's approval to continue. Recently pharmacies are soliciting permission to provide refills for three months. Once permission is received, it will continue. Often the prescribed person does not understand the consequences.

Also, some pharmacies, especially mail order stores, will automatically refill three- or six-months' worth of medications at a time and bill insurance then charge a credit card that is on file for any difference or co-pay. Good luck trying to get a refund!

Making a list and what to do

Verify with the primary physician what medications are valid and should be taken. Take this list with you to the pharmacy. Also take the current physician summary, POA, health surrogate/directive and the patient with you. It is best to have the patient with you if at all possible. Ask to speak with the pharmacist to update the pharmacy records regarding what medications will no longer be available for refills by the patient. They should comply, if not ask for the Manager. Once complete and verified that no other prescriptions will be filled other than the current medications, insist that these medications only be refilled for 30 days at a time. Whenever a medication is discontinued communicate the change with the pharmacy. This step is paramount!

Make a dispensing list of medications

In Chapter 13 "Organizational Notebook Explained" section there is a Medication List form that can be used and updated. This list can also be helpful for the person you are taking care of because it provides a list of current meds with a name, a sample of the pill be taped on the space provided to show what the pill looks like, dosage (how much should be taken), and when it should be taken. There is also a place that gives special instructions such as take with food, take on empty stomach, do not take with other meds, etc. Also, important information about the last refill and the number of pills purchased. This information in particular can be extremely important if the medication is not in a dispenser or if the medication is a controlled substance that needs to be monitored. Closely monitoring controlled substances is for everyone's benefit.

All medication lists should be updated each time a prescription is changed in any way. Often prescriptions may be reduced or even discontinued. If multiple people are helping with caregiving, all should be aware of any changes immediately. The patient may disagree because a specific medication has been a part of their routine, but it is important to reinforce what is written in the discharge notes from the physician's office or healthcare facility. This is the number one reason to keep them handy and updated in the Organization Paperwork notebook!

Pre-Packaging

A pros-cons about Pre-Package medications: These are bubble type pre-packed dosages of medications. This can be great regarding ease of use, but when medications change, all previous packages must be discarded. This is for safety. Sadly, it is a waste of money especially when some medications cost $1 or more per dose.

Using a dispensing device

If using a dispensing device, the "medication list" is an important guideline to refill the device properly with updated medications and dispensing information. Also, when choosing a dispensing device there are a few things to consider.

Managing a dispensing device. Who is refilling the device?

If a nurse is in charge of refilling a dispenser it is important to communicate the most current medication information ahead of the visit. Otherwise, the nurse may have outdated information and refill according to outdated information. Make sure all medications have been refilled so that the dispenser can be completely filled. If the medications are not available, the nurse cannot partially refill due to potentially not having the correct dosage or medication available for the entire term.

If the caregiver is refilling the device always make sure to refill completely. Never partially refill with the idea that later whatever medications were not available will be added. This can be an extremely dangerous situation and easily overlooked with everything that needs to be accomplished as a caregiver.

What kind of devices are available?

Here is a list of devices that can be purchased. Depending on the price point that you are comfortable spending, a 30-day dispenser is often the most easily used and only needs attention once a month. The following dispensers are in order of capacity and preference. The website address is provided for specific products if not available on a common online service such as Amazon.

Hero smart dispenser. PRO: This is an ingenious self-dispensing machine which holds 90 days' worth of medications. This is a personal favorite because it not only blinks when it is time to take a medication, but one-button pushed, sorts and dispenses the dose. It also has a special feature though an app for cell phones that alerts the caregiver if the medication has not been dispensed. If it is long distance or local, a caregiver can remind the person to go and take their medication. It is a one-year minimum service subscription or an upfront option payment, both include the dispensing machine. CON: This device can only dispense whole pills. This did not work for me since a ½ tablet was needed. The company was very understanding and accepted cancellation and acknowledged the issue.   PURCHASE OPTION: www.Herohealth.com

Med-E-Lert, Locking 28-Day Automatic Pill Dispenser. PRO: This dispenser locks and only allows current day medication to be dispensed. A reminder time and alert (three tone choices) can be set. CON: Only holds 28 days of medication. Attention to battery life is important. PURCHASE OPTION: This device can be purchased on Amazon.

31 Day Pill Box by MEDca. PRO: This dispenser has a slot for 'today's pill' box compartment. Then the dispenser box compartment can be put back in its slot upside down when the day is complete and empty. It is completely manual. The days are printed in large numbers, so it is easy to read. The dispenser is round and easy to see wherever stored. The 31 days are suitable for each month days whether 28, 29, 30, or 31.

CON: Feels a little larger than most manual dispensers. No locking device. PURCHASE OPTION: Can be purchased on Amazon.

The Original Monthly Medication Organizer by MEDCENTER Systems. PRO: This model comes with or without an Easy Set Reminder Clock. It holds 31 days' worth of medications and has a 'Today's Pills' tray. CON: Attention must be paid to the battery life. Dispensing is manual. No locking device. PURCHASE OPTION: Can be purchased on Amazon.

There are literally hundreds of variations of medication organization and dispensing devices. These reviews are a few that through experience worked very well or have good potential. Products come and go; these are items that were available when this book was published. Updated items may appear or disappear in future printings. For an easy access to these products you can visit gauntletofcaregiving.com

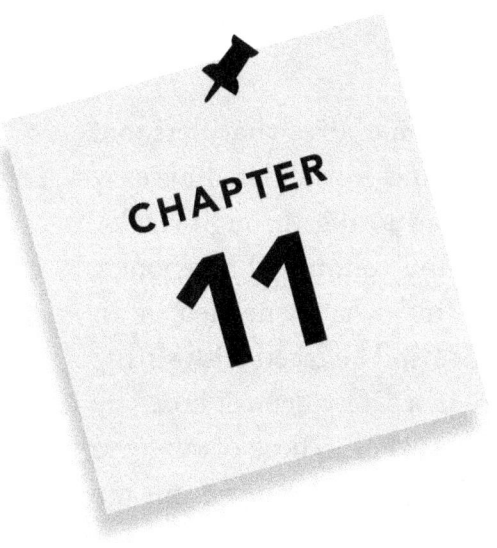

How To Organize Everyday Paperwork

FROM THIS ...

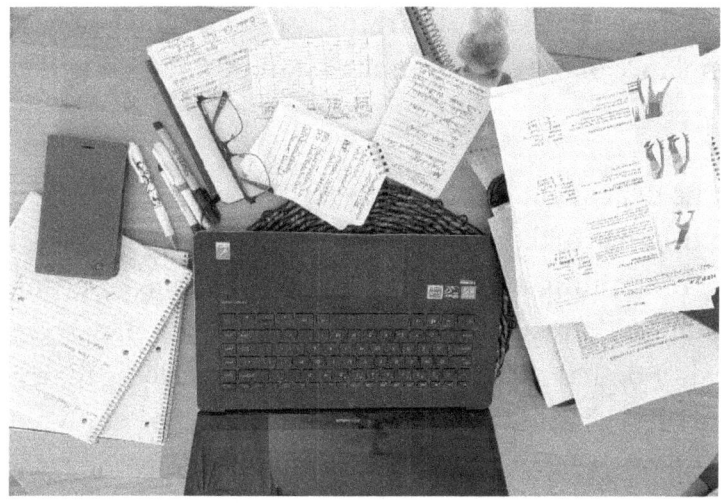

TO THIS!

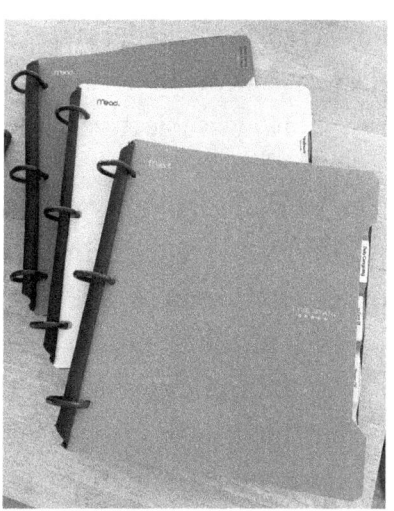

How to Organize Everyday Paperwork – Part 1

To Organize – Or Not – There is no singular answer! The "Data Dump Gauntlet" in Chapter 5 requires diligence and being organized can help. By now this Gauntlet is a very real nemesis if you have begun helping someone else. As you read this section and possibly glaze over, stay with it. Once accomplished it will be a huge responsibility off your endless list of tasks and reduce many aspects of the gauntlet. What a concept, right!?!

Although somewhat repetitive in this presentation, it is imperative that personal information about the person you are caring for is located and consolidated for easy accessibility. Ask anyone who has been a caregiver and had to dig through stacks, drawers, boxes and filing cabinets full of papers, toted around volumes of notebooks, folders, and papers in bags. Or what it is like to try to find what is needed in an emergency even in someone else's organized home or office and be faced with sifting through all of these places just to find out documents are in a safety deposit box, safe not knowing the combo, or with an attorney and it is the weekend. Those of you who have done this, you are my soulmates. I have written about this not just from my experiences but also from similar and shared experiences.

During the process of writing "The Gauntlet of Caregiving," it has become apparent to me that everyone organizes in a unique way. There are people who have piles of papers on their desk, on countertops, boxes, you name it. To someone else it may look like chaos, to the owner every paper has its place. For me it has depended on the decade, the job, and expectations of the industry how paperwork, either tangible or digital, should be categorized, filed, cataloged, or stored. For the most part in my lifestyle and business there has always been some assemblance of organization, at least in my opinion which is not always subjective.

The workable filing system must be dependent on the material. Artwork such as you would find in publishing is filed differently than a filing system found in a medical office environment, a legal office, or a billing department. In our digital age, setting up files in the cloud, on a computer, backup storage, laptop, or cell device may seem easier than piles of papers. In reality digital files are not completely different than a paper file drawer system. Files are files, whether digital or paper. All can be cluttered whether on a counter, on a computer screen or buried deep within the memory of a terabyte of disc storage space. Where you store personal files is always up to the user. No matter what anyone says, your home and with its devices is your castle, not even the digital software on a computer with automatic suggestions that need to be applied to filing are written in stone. If you do a search online there are classes to teach how to organize digital files. Yes, this is a thing, and you will pay to acquire this knowledge! So, never forget YOU can decide how to organize documents in your own castle.

A big BUT here! When files are someone else's personal information it is a different story! I do not have statistics, but it is apparent that Baby boomers are the first generation to store more documents in a digital format than previously in history. Documents also are often duplicated in a paper form and filed away, somewhere. As a digital lover, much to my personal dismay as a caregiver, discovering that paper files are the most user friendly and easily accessible was a huge surprise.

Don't totally discard using the digital devices. Using a smart phone as a backup for scheduled calendar dates is useful especially if you are not living with the person full time as a caregiver to have access to the paper calendar. Using the notification feature can help with preparing for the event by using the settings available on the electronic calendar. A great feature for the caregiver to use. It is not recommended to take pictures of any personal health information and store it on a device. If you insist it is important for the safety and security of information to learn how to use "lock" on the documents saved on your electronic device. Cell phone photos can be accessed if someone hacks your phone security. All phones have what are called "notes," and instructions on how to store information and secure it within notes can be researched. With an industry of organized fraud and the need for 2F-Authentication, locking files is imperative.

Producing a filing and organizing system for caregiving has much to do with what is required for the end result. Ease of transport, ease of locating information, and ease of updating. Not necessarily in this order. Discovering how and what needs to be easily accessible and portable without the need for internet or cell signal was to say the least, mind boggling. Through trial and error, a simple binder with paper copies of documents, note sheets, and important personal information, organized with easy to find categories was, much to my chagrin, the ultimate answer. The" Organizational Notebook" instructions in Part 2 of "How to Organize Everyday Paperwork" fulfill this niche.

Within "How to Organize Everyday Paperwork - Part 2" information is included about how to take notes, set reminders, keep a calendar, and create a notebook. As stated before, being organized, and filing important documents/information is a very personal issue for everyone. Often the biggest challenge is to find what you need. Acknowledgement that another persons' system is a best kept secret and sometimes needs deciphering with almost military skill by an outsider, will be helpful. Personal information is a very delicate subject for the person who needs to depend on a caregiver no matter your current or prior relationship.

When asking for personal information, proceed with caution and compassion. Until someone has needed help, he/she has been self-sufficient their entire lives. This would be the same if you ever choose to help a friend or family member, especially aging parents. DO NOT go digging through drawers, filing cabinets, or anywhere unless you receive permission and discuss this with the person you are helping first. Repercussions will happen and often it establishes a distrustful environment if the need for knowledge supersedes the consideration of getting permission to invade his/her privacy. Every time you need to go digging, ask. Yes, it is repetitive, but it is the right thing to do. With regards to a spouse or other family member who may have moved in with you, have a conversation with them and do the information gathering process together.

Providing children or loved ones with the location of information in case of emergency is good practice. The location of information can be stored on an electronic device to be referenced if the need arises. Make sure not to label specifically on a digital device without a passcode. For example, do not type; Bank Account at ABC Bank, account number 123456, username Andy, password Andy123456. You get it, right?

The acronym ICE (In Case of Emergency) is generally recognized by emergency responders for essential information or personal contact if needed. Provide a password or code for a person you trust to access this on your electronic device. Record this information on the "Username and Passwords" form which is available in the Appendix section or order on the website. Store this form in the Green "Confidential Estate and Legal" notebook and keep it in a secure place such as a safe. Programs such as Excel and Adobe Acrobat can be password protected if using electronic files. Remember, if you are incapacitated without prior plans for someone else to have access to devices and pass coded documents, no one will be able to help.

Note: A DNR on the refrigerator may supersede any Healthcare Directive paperwork that cannot be accessed in an emergency. Make sure this is understood!

What not to do is as important as what you do!

It is not advisable to walk into any situation and try to re-organize someone else's world. The need to do this is well meaning and well-intended to make your life a bit less stressful. But it sets up a scenario for many stressful emotional issues for the person you ultimately want to help. Instead use the information within Part 2 of this section to help you organize what is needed as a Caregiver. Asking permission to put together an "Organizational Notebook" as a onetime project so that you can help when needed can be met with appreciation and understanding. But in some situations it may not, so patience is the best way to gently put it aside.

If the suggestion of collecting personal information is not met with cooperation, the information can be gathered over time. My recommendation is to become an observer.

Organize yourself, not the one you are taking care of. Become a chameleon with the ability to transform into using the current way of seeing and organizing his/her world and maintain it for them. With "The Essentials List" you will know what information is important and can make copies or take pictures of the items as they are located to include in the "Organizational Notebooks." Pay attention to where documents are located and note on the "Essentials List Location" form. Become aware that making copies of some documents is against Federal law. Read documents carefully!

A Mom Moment: When growing up in order to help me be more understanding of other people rather than judgmental, mom would say to me, "Put yourself in their shoes for a day." I am sure she hoped to instill empathy in my youthful smugness. This is an old saying, but for a caregiver the idea of "Putting yourself in their shoes for a day" can be instrumental in learning how to help someone else.

Takeaways:

- Part 2 and Part 3 are essential for organizing "The Data Dump Gauntlet" information.
- Security is paramount for personal information, usernames, passwords, and legal documents.
- Proceed with kindness and compassion. Put yourself in their position...

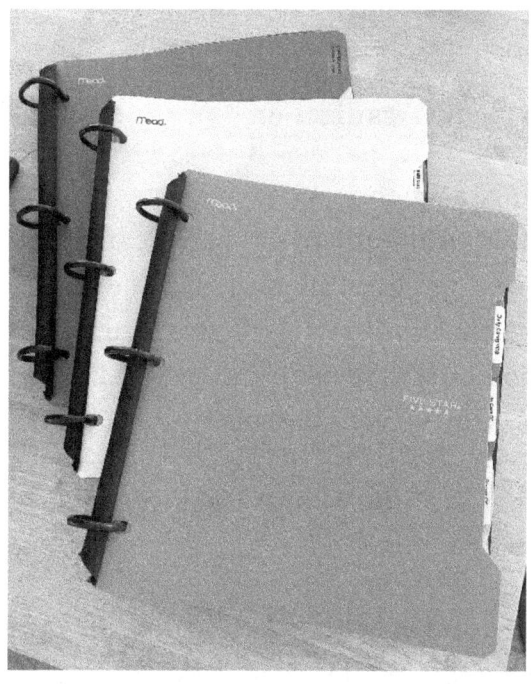

How To Organize Everyday Paperwork-Part 2

From chaotic piles, boxes and bags of folders, papers, and notes, to a peaceful simple three notebook system.

Why would I want so much paperwork?

Why can't everything be done online?

With technology and portals, why have paperwork? One particularly important reason. After much trial and error, having all information easily to grab and go is paramount. When there are multiple people taking care of one person, communication in writing can mean the difference in life and death. Yes, this is the truth! Ask yourself this question; "If I became incapacitated today, who would know my doctors name, who would I want to make decisions for my healthcare, who knows about wishes if I cannot make decisions for myself?" Then ask yourself about your elderly parents; "Where do I find the Power of Attorney, the Estate Planning paperwork, the Trust documents, who is the Trustee, who is their doctor, what do they eat for breakfast, who are their friends or affiliations?"

The simple answer is all this information can be placed into one convenient compact resource, printed and included in the three "Organizational Notebooks." No more need for confusion or guess work, multiple portals, multiple places to seek information, or a list of digital usernames or passwords for a simple task!

Nuts and Bolts of Document Organization

Organization of anything, as mentioned previously, is often predetermined by the situation. Documents that are required by healthcare, financial and Government institutions are ever changing. For this reason, "The Gauntlet of Caregiving" will continue to update this publication in its electronic format. It is encouraged for readers to return and check periodically to review what may be updated with changes to forms and information that meets new requirements.

Organizational Notebook – What is an Organizational Notebook and why is it important?

You can't carry a filing cabinet with you and not all information can be found online in one place. Hopefully by now you have an idea of how important it is to have all personal information at your fingertips. If not, it is my fault, so here is more explanation. This notebook should include all the information listed here along with any additional information that is important. Notations are made when an item should be kept with a third party or separately from the Organizational Notebook. There are recommendations along the way to help you figure out what to do with confidential and security risk items.

The forms and organizational pages can be previewed in the back of this book. A pre-printed compilation of this Organizational Notebook, with a binder, may be available for purchase at a later date. Packets of forms can be purchased. If you are interested, visit the website gauntletofcaregiving.com.

The information is organized in three different notebooks. There is an expanded explanation to follow which will guide you through each section and how it is used. This chapter can be used as a checklist, it will speed up the process of what to keep in the "Organizational Notebooks."

Notebook number one used for daily use. (See chapter 12, Binders and Such for info on Purple notebook) This notebook includes the following:

- Calendar/Schedule

- Medication List

- Daily Caregiving Notes

- Healthcare Directive and DNR (Copies)

- In Case of Emergency information sheet

- Power of Attorney (copy)

- Important Personal Information List (Use this sheet to gather information & check list)

Notebook number two is set up and organized to easily take it with you to appointments and contains information needed by healthcare providers. (See chapter 12, Binders and Such for info on White notebook) Also, this notebook will provide you with healthcare information across institutions in one easy to reference location.

This includes the following:

- Health information (A comprehensive questionnaire regarding health Q&A)

- Healthcare Records (Visit summaries and notes)

- Physician Information (Primary and Specialty Physicians information)

- Nursing Home/Rehab (When someone has been admitted to hospital and sent to Rehab)

- Veterans Administration

- DME Medical Equipment information sheets

- Appointment notes blank sheets.

Notebook number three is for confidential information and should be kept in a safe, secure place and only key people know where it is located. (See chapter 12, Binders and Such for info on notebook) This book includes the following:

- Attorney/Accountant information (includes documents held & by whom)

- Power of Attorney (Original & extra copies)

- Personal Financial Documents

- Estate Planning

- Security Codes, User ID's, and Passwords

Again, binder recommendations can be found in Chapter 12 "Binders and Such." This is a review of options and recommendations.

Part 3 of "How to Organize Everyday Paperwork" has an expanded explanation of each section of the three notebooks and what paperwork should be included in the specifically labeled section.

The initial task of getting organized may seem tedious, boring, and possibly confusing. By following the information here, one label at a time from beginning to end, the daunting task of organization will prove much simpler than gathering the very important information needed in preparation to be organized. This process will also end the hunting and digging to find a document or information that is needed immediately.

Hang in there! When complete, this part of the Gauntlet will prove to be very satisfying, and a huge stress relief for all involved. Once done the notebooks only need to be updated with new or changed information.

How To Organize Everyday Paperwork-Part 3

From chaotic piles, boxes and bags of folders, papers and notes, to a peaceful simple three notebook system.

When thinking about personal information, the first thought most people have is that it is no one else's business. This is true, laws have been written to protect individual rights to keep personal, financial and health information private. But... and this is a big but, someone, at some time, will need to know what is kept where. This need will be if or when a person needs help, if or when a person must liquidate assets in order to pay for help and ultimately when a person is no longer with us.

These three books talked about here will have a great impact on all of these needs. The best laid plans can often create a labyrinth to navigate when it comes to a lifetime spent living and accumulating. History is riddled with stories of misplaced documents such as a will, title, and money. When illness is involved, there are terrible instances of malfeasance. Facing the fact that anyone who has not shared who their attorney is, which bank they use, who planned their estate, who their doctor is, and more is a concern that needs to be addressed.

The concept of these books is not just an overzealous desire to organize, but an effort to create a tool to help a person in need in a compassionate, empathic, and loving way by the loved one and caregiver.

Professional facilities have set standards for care. They are required to keep limited important personal information about their residents in a central secure place to be accessed if an emergency arises. There are more people wanting to stay at home, needing help when the time comes to move into the next level of care, so there is a greater need for important information to be accessible for friends and family caregivers.

Notebook #1 - The Purple Binder

This binder can help to make the person you care for more comfortable in time. At first the change may be a bit daunting. But the simplicity, once in use, will become a go to place for confirmation and communication for everyone involved in caregiving. It includes a calendar, so everyone knows what is happening on each day. The daily routine form is used to understand individual preferences to help lessen stress of "Merging Lifestyles" and is useful for communication when professional caregivers or "Respite Care" support is used. It also provides one place to find in-case-of-emergency information.

Pre-Tabs: Basic information sheet - For some this form may seem useless or redundant, especially if a person knows the information already. Placing this sheet in front of this notebook provides anyone, when in an emergency situation, an easy reference. The form lists the residential address, the closest physical crossroads which EMS will ask for, and caregiver/case manager information.

Tab 1: Calendar & Schedule – A paper calendar can be downloaded from several sources online or get a free one from your local merchant. For a daily calendar that is printed with the current year and dates, the Microsoft program Word and Google Calendar can produce monthly blanks that can be downloaded and printed on your own printer and 3-holed punched to fit in the notebook. If you choose to buy one, make sure it will fit into the 3-ring binder of choice and can be 3-holed punched.

In Chapter 12, "Binders and Such" there are recommendations for the make and model of recommended binders. After much experimentation, a three-ring binder is preferable because documents can be easily added and moved around.

Tab 2: Daily Routine Notes - First insert medication list, then notes after.

List of Current Medications form. This list is for daily reference. It includes Name of medication, dosage, dosage instructions, a place to tape a sample pill so the receiver can see what he/she is taking if interested, Prescribing Doctor, Reason for medication. (Have copies in both Notebook 1 & 2, make a habit of updating in book 1, then copy for book 2. This form should be kept up to date and it is IMPORTANT to cross through old information!)

Daily Routine Notes (For easy reference, chronological is recommended with most recent notes first.) When taking care of someone at home with or without the help of professional caregivers, this form can be so helpful when other family members or professionals provide respite care! No guessing about how someone likes their coffee, when he/she eats lunch and what is preferred to eat, and so on. Having a journal of entries to refer back to is not only helpful for all concerned, but especially for a physician visit! Being able to tell a doctor, this happened a week ago on this date and again on this date, can make a huge difference in treatment for acute or chronic physical and mental health issues.

Tab 3: In Case of Emergency (ICE) - This section is paramount! If an emergency happens no one needs to wonder where to find numbers of who else to contact after EMS has been called.

Compiling a list can be short, offering to give the major contacts an extended list is helpful or can be included in this section. As mentioned in the "Welcome to the Gauntlet," in the past it was common for all this information to be in a specific place, usually the inside front cover of the printed phone book. These days with digital files, smart phones, and computers, who knows where to find information? Here is the place!

A copy of the DNR, Health Surrogate & Healthcare Directive should also be placed in this section for easy reference. This is important for several reasons; first so that there is a written wish list, second if a DNR is posted on a refrigerator the EMS personnel may or may not resuscitate without direction from the designated person which is in written form, also it is important to know the wishes of the patient and the authority of the Health Care Surrogate. Including a signed DNR form, Health Surrogate/Healthcare Directive/Healthcare POA will answer any questions health care professionals need to proceed quickly! Note: Fivewishes.org has a healthcare directive information booklet and forms available for a small fee (at time of writing less than $5-$15.00) and are specific for each State or ask your healthcare provider, they sometimes offer them for free.

Tab 4: Power of Attorney - It is important to have a copy of the POA in this folder for easy access. The person(s) listed on the in case of emergency information should correspond with the name(s) on this document for the safety of the patient. The original should be placed in notebook three and kept in a safe place.

Tab 5: Important Personal Information list – This is the basic list of what should be located to have when needed. It can be checked off. Also this same list is duplicated with added blanks and referred to as the "Locator List of Essential Information." With permission, this list can be included in any notebook. For security purposes and peace of mind, make sure that all copies of the locator list are updated and replaced when changes are made.

Notebook #2 - The White Binder

This is your GO TO notebook for doctor appointments. One notebook with all the history in one place. Copies of ID's, insurance cards, and other items can be invaluable to have with you just in case the originals are not handy. This is healthcare history and information at your fingertips. Be diligent about using the appointment note pages and this notebook will always be up to date. Keep records in chronological order with the most recent on top for easy reference. Each heading has a divider that separates the sections. Forms and other documents can be found in Chapter 13 "Organizational Notebook Downloads."

NOTE: Ask for business cards and tape them to the page that identifies the provider, don't be shy. You will be happy you asked later. :)

Tab 1: Important Personal Information – Often the person you are providing care for will have the following items in their wallet or purse. Having copies available in the binder will help to expedite filling out paperwork when needed. If for some reason one of these items is lost, having a copy is helpful to know the information needed when requesting a new or duplicate copy. In most situations the original needs to be present when an ID is requested. (Note: A wallet or purse is a very personal item that should be treated with respect. Always ask for access!)

Identifications - Make copies for this folder, keep originals with owner.
Driver's License(s) or State Issued ID**
Social Security Card(s)
Birth Certificate
Proof of Citizenship or Green card
Passport
Veteran: DD214
Pension Identification Card(s)

NOTE** - Important information: For anyone who no longer drives but holds a driver's license. There is an expiration date on every driver's license. A State ID must be requested to replace a driver's license PRIOR TO EXPIRATION! Ask me how I know.

This is a challenge because a government office, Notary or any financial institution will not honor an expired driver's license as identification! The transition of a Driver's License to State ID in most States can be done online and a new State ID mailed. Check online for the state of issuance and for other required identification that may be needed to accomplish this. There most likely will be a cost involved.

> **NOTE: Important information: Photocopying any U.S. government identification is a violation of Title 18, US Code Part 1, Chapter 33, Section 701 –www.defense.gov*
>
> *This pertains to military members, their families, and Defense Department employees. The result of photocopying these ID's can be a fine or imprisonment. It is recommended these IDs remain in the possession of the person and a caregiver should know where to find the ID when needed.*

Personal Health Information – Gather, make copies and/or record location.
Insurances, Directives and Healthcare Records/Providers
Medicare Card(s)
Supplemental Health Insurance Cards (Copy front & back)
Long Term Health Care Insurance
Dental & Vision Insurance
Other Health Plans such as VA Enrollee, Government Employee, or Pension Plans (Do not copy Government ID's especially Military ID's)**
Copy of current list of Medications from Book 1 (Have copies in both Notebook 1 & 2, make a habit of updating in book 1, then copy for book 2. This form should be kept up to date!
Current Doctors or Specialty Care Physician(s) forms
List of Hospital visited and current status forms.
Health History form completed.
Living Will copy.
Healthcare Directive copy.
Healthcare Surrogate Designation copy.
Healthcare Power of Attorney copy.

Tab 2: Healthcare Records - This section includes discharge paperwork from any healthcare provider, notes from physician appointments, phone calls, acute care medical notes when issues arise, Caregiver notes for daily awareness of issues that arise and solutions that worked.

Tab 3: Physician Information Form - (Tape the Business Card here or fill in the form for each) Placing these forms in the folder can be in alphabetical by name or type of doctor such as Primary Physician, Pulmonary Physician, Eye Doctor, Eye specialist, Physical or Occupational Therapist, Cardiologist, Oncologist, Rheumatologist, etc.

Categorize any Physician other than primary doctors in Specialty Physician Healthcare. (Example: Eye Care Specialist such as an Ophthalmologist is an Eye Doctor and often performs cataract surgery, he/she would be categorized as a Specialty Physician or a doctor that is seen for a specialty not on a regular basis possibly annually.) It is important to keep these separated to know who is seen on a regular basis. Sometimes a pulmonary or cardiologist is seen on a regular basis and should be included as a Primary. If only seen once, it would be categorized as a Specialty Physician. Why is this important? If the person you care for goes into an independent, assistant, or long-term care facility this information is required to be on file! They will be contacting the physicians for checkups and updates, and without separation an office visit may not be necessary. Having the results of a one-time visit vs regular required visits will make the process much smoother and less stressful for everyone, especially the patient!

Specialty Physician Healthcare Forms - (Tape the Business Card here and fill in form for each specialty physician making sure to include healthcare facility information)

Example: Cancer Treatment Facility. This would be a separate category for easy reference. Sometimes specialty care is being conducted along with other Physician appointments and can be confusing when tossed in with the others. Also having its own category makes it stand out and helpful when in the middle of a situation it acts as a reminder… "oh wait, we need to consult with blah blah, the Oncologists before doing whatever…"

Suggested Treatments and Physicians for this "Specialty Physician" category would be Urology, Nephrology, Oncology/Cancer Treatment, Radiology Cancer Treatment, Cancer Surgical treatments, etc. Notes about the current status of the treatment are important to keep up to date.

Tab 4: Hospital Information Form - (Tape the Business Card here and fill in form for each) Chronological Order works best for Hospitals. The list provides for multiple visits to the same hospital. If a person had a major surgery years ago, make a note on the information sheet of what was done, where it was done, and dates. This will help to fill out the Personal Information Form where you can reference history quickly. Why? Do you remember where you had your tonsils or appendix out, how old were you?

Tab 5: Veterans' Health Information - (Tape the Business Card here and fill in form for each). There are many different departments in the VA Administration. Alphabetical works good here, then chronological within the subheads. A VA hospital Doctor is different than a VA Clinic Doctor. When using VA physicians and community physicians it can become very confusing with regard to visits and especially prescriptions! If a veteran has been enrolled with the VA healthcare system, he/she will have an identification card that states the person is a "VA Healthcare Enrollee." When refilling prescriptions it is important to know where the Physician is employed. Also keeping all physicians informed of medications and treatments is best practice for safe caregiving.

Tab 6: Nursing Home Information Form - (Tape the Business Card here and fill in form for each). Chronological Order works for this when a stay is for rehabilitation. Permanent Addresses which have changed from Independent to Assisted to Nursing Home Care can be by date, A-Z, or whatever makes sense to you.

Tab 7: DME Medical Equipment: (It is rare the delivery personnel provide a business card, but there should be an identifying sticker on the equipment) ME/Medical Equipment List and Providers Durable Medical Equipment or DME is a term that references items such as medical supplies, walkers, wheelchairs, oxygen equipment, etc., that is covered by insurance and provided by a local vendor. Some equipment is rented and requires contact with the vendor if a physician's order changes. Example: When a patient changes status from walker to wheelchair and should not use a walker, the walker should be returned to the vendor otherwise the patient could be charged a monthly rental fee once insurance receives new orders for a wheelchair. Often the pickup of equipment is the responsibility of the patient. This happens often and the patient is stuck paying for equipment not used.

Be aware these days a simple walker could involve two or three companies. Yes, this is crazy and true. A fulfillment company, a billing company, a delivery company and potentially another delivery company! This makes keeping track of medical equipment even more important. If the billing company is not notified of any change, they will begin to bill the patient when insurance is cancelled. All parties need to be notified that orders have been changed and the equipment is no longer needed. Document all conversations, if you do not, it will cost money. Seriously! As a caregiver there can be situations it could be passed on to you for failure to communicate with all parties including family members, conservators, and guardians.

Tab 8: Appointment Note Blanks – These blanks are used to take notes for appointments and would be included with summary of visit provided by healthcare facility and placed in the Health Care Records section.

Notebook #3 - Green Notebook

Locator List of Essential Information form

Fill out this form which is the same list of "Personal Information" with added blank spaces to help with locating items if not stored in these books. Place it in the front of this notebook.

Attorney & Accountant - Originals

Attorney and Accountant information is a particularly important financial section. Often documents such as a Power of Attorney, Last Will and Testament, Trusts, and others are not kept at home but stored with the Attorney who created them. The form with location of documents is important. Too often documents are scattered in different locations and sometimes not found when their information could be extremely helpful.

Power of Attorney - Originals

This is where the originals can be kept if not located in an Attorney's office. If these documents are located elsewhere, a notation should be made and a copy of the POA kept here for reference. A copy of the POA should also be kept in Notebook 1 and 2 for reference. Originals can be later provided to an institution upon request.

Personal Financial – List location of originals

There are four sections: Personal Financial Liabilities (Bills), Personal Financial Income and Sources, Personal Financial Assets (Owned), Personal Financial Businesses/ LLC/etc.

Motor Vehicle Registration or Title (Cars, Campers, Motorcycle, Mobile Homes) If financed, Financial Institution information, copy of loan(s) & Payment Information

Income Verification from ALL sources including Pension Benefits

Checking/Savings, Brokerage accounts, Statements of all for past 3-6 months

Income Tax Filing for last 5 yrs.

Mortgage Information (Asset Liability Form)

Property Tax Bill(s) & Addresses (The property address does not always appear on the bill)

Property Insurance Providers (Homeowners, Vehicle, Boat, Camper, Golf Cart, Motorcycle, etc.)

Personal Residence and Value (Required for Government programs that are based on assets and income such as Medicaid, County/City in Home Care, & other programs)

The first question to come to mind when reviewing this list is "Why does anyone other than me need this information? It is no one else's business!" Well, usually no one, but these documents will be required when seeking the use of services from a County or State care program providing nurses and caregivers or Medicaid benefits.

Usernames and Passwords

Username and Passwords can be in a written list in the Organizational Notebook number three, but for security reasons as with all information in this notebook, it should be stored in a secure place such as a safe or with an Attorney.

Usernames and passwords can be kept in an Excel file with a password for protection. You can keep the password written on this form in the notebook. If you file it discretely somewhere else, be careful and it is not suggested. Discretely means DO NOT LABEL what it is. If needed give it to someone else just in case you forget it but be cognizant that it could be lost or used maliciously if found by someone else. It is not recommended you allow any electronic device to automatically store usernames and passwords.

Sometimes passwords change, keeping the paper record up to date will be advantageous. If designated, someone with a Power of Attorney may be able to access an account without the password. Do not rely on this though. Increasingly it is more difficult to use a POA for this purpose quickly, even stopping an existing cable/internet account can become a challenge! It is easier to have the person you care for give permission to a vendor to speak to you by phone than to do it yourself with a POA! An example, switching cable/internet companies will require the owner to give permission to speak with you! Crazy but true.

Cell Phone Organization

Be incredibly careful carrying documents on your cell phone. With a username and password it is possible to keep information somewhat safe. I have done it using PDF documents, links to secure cloud storage, and photos of documents. After fumbling around, trying to access the internet or cell phone service inside of healthcare facilities. It quickly became apparent that electronic devices are inherently dependent on signals that are often, if not always, blocked within healthcare facilities when you need information the most.

Photos work well but are not secure. Use photos at your own risk. Every state has laws concerning photos of licenses and government issued ID's that are not your own, just like the any law, DO YOUR RESEARCH. It is handy to have a picture of items which will be easily accessible on your smartphone. But it is not recommended.

Is Photocopying Government ID's Illegal?

YES. More information at the government website: www.defense.gov

---

Reminder: Ask for a business card everywhere you go! If there is no business card, write information on the form including the name of the person you have communicated with about the subject. This is especially important for future reference. Did I mention how important this is? Doing this will help keep everyone informed, and the person who is receiving care safer.

Binders and Such

Oh, for the love of binders! Said no one?

This review is based mostly on experience and research for a solution that is as simple as organizing electronic files on a computer. Well, almost, this isn't an option to randomly search for a document but can be considered the next best thing.

When seeking a binder, the main goal was to find pieces that were easily adaptable to the duty of caregiving without having to order expensive customized components. If demand requests a customized solution in the future, it may be considered. For now, all the components can be easily purchased online and delivered to your home, which when caregiving for someone else, this convenience makes life easier!

So, here we go with what has been found to meet the criteria of low cost, flexibility of use, lightweight and easily portable, yet durable enough to withstand daily use and abuse. That is within reason.

Binders:

Spiral bound vs three ring binders.

Spiral binders offer the option to have file folders with pockets just as other binders, the setup is easy, but to customize and change pages is a challenge and became more of an adaptation to the preset organizing of the binder itself.

After much experimentation, three ring binders win as the most flexible to keep paperwork organized and changeable. But there are so many different types of three ring binders, it is possible you have many laying around that you can use. That would be ok, but hard side binders can be heavy, bulky and cumbersome for daily use. These were the initial choices until a better solution was found.

WINNER! A flexible binder made by Mead in their FIVE STAR FLEX line 1" binder customizable hybrid notebook binder. This front pocket allows for use of a custom cover sheet to identify each book and is refillable, made by ACCO.

These binders can be purchased online at Amazon or most office supply websites. The cost is a little more expensive than a standard hard cover three ring binder, but it's flexibility to organize, expand and update along with its portfolio fold over feature has become the go to binder for The Gauntlet of Caregiving Organizational Notebooks.

The binders come in a nice selection of colors so each "Organizational Notebook" can be a different color. Color coding is one of the easiest ways to communicate functionality for what an item is used to perform. For this reason, three different colors have been chosen.

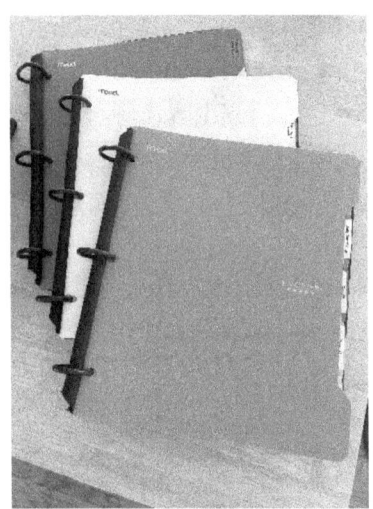

Purple for daily use.

White for important health care information.

Green for secure financial documents.

The only notebook that does not come in a customizable cover is the Green notebook. For security purposes this works out well. Only those who should be in the know will recognize it for what it is. A cover sheet on the inside can identify the owner if there is more than one person in a family or residence. One financial notebook can be used for multiple people if accounts are in all names. Otherwise the information contained in the notebook identifies the person to whom it belongs.

Internal tabs and pockets

Often the way to organize documents is a personal preference whether in a file drawer, in a binder or on a computer. These notebooks are set up for a specific purpose, this is why the tabs and tab folders are so very important in the organization of these notebooks. Again, much research and experimentation has been done to produce a workable solution for caregiving communication and organization.

Each binder uses a different set of tab sheets. These sheets can be purchased online at Amazon or at most office supply websites. Notebook one uses 5-Tabs, Notebooks two and three use 8-tabs.

Here is a list of the tabs used.

Purple Book:
Calendar/Schedule
Daily Caregiver Notes
In Case of Emergency
Power of Attorney (Copy)

White Book:
Personal Health Information
Healthcare Records
Physician Information
Hospital Information
Nursing Home/Rehab Information
Veterans Administration
DME Medical Equipment
Appointment Notes – Blanks

Green Book:
Attorney & Accountant
Power of Attorney (Original or its location)
Personal Financial
Estate Planning (Documents or where to find)
Security UID & PW (User Identification and Password List)
Final Arrangements
Last Will and Testament (Or its location)
Miscellaneous Original Documents (Such as Healthcare Directives, copies should be in Purple book)

Organizational
Notebooks Explained

Welcome to the document and forms download page.

These are documents and forms that are in PDF format. If you wish to download these documents, go to the website: gauntletofcaregiving.com for more information. There are also document samples in the appendix section of the publication.

Because this subject is ever evolving and the Legal, Healthcare and Government continue to protect us, these documents and forms will change from time to time. I recommend you look at the date posted and do your own due diligence through whatever source you use to confirm that the form you use from this format is the most up to date available. - End of Disclaimer

This is where the organization experience begins. This will be the least expensive way to get organized for caregiving. Chapter 11 "How To Organize Everyday Paperwork" provides expanded information about how to use the documents that go in each of the "Organizational Paperwork" notebooks. There are form examples printed in the back of this book, but unless this is the most recent revision of printing the forms may be outdated and should only be used as examples.

All downloads are in PDF format. Before printing read the following:

These forms can be printed on normal printer paper, 3-hole punched or whatever the printer requires for the notebook tabs.

3-hole punch paper requires correct orientation for the printer and the PDF's do not adjust, so the operator must know the printer requirements.

When printing, if a document is more than one page, it can be printed on two sides if the printer allows for two-sided printing. If not, each form page will be one-sided. For example: a six-page document printed on both sides will be three sheets of paper. If printed on one side, it will be 6 pages.

KNOW YOUR PRINTER! You can waste time and money if you do not. If this project seems overwhelming, you may order pre-printed forms and tabs (with instructional information imprinted) from the same vendor you used to purchase this book.

Why has this information been made available? Many people are very much do it yourselfers and I relate! So this chapter is dedicated to those who prefer the freedom to do it their way. But a fair option for most people is to purchase the pre-printed forms and tabs and place them in your choice of three-ring binder or purchase the suggested notebooks provided within this chapter.

How To Organize Everyday Paperwork Labels – This sheet of labels will assist to complete the "Organizational Paperwork" folder tabs. These tab labels are in PDF format and can be downloaded to print on Avery Easy Peel Label stock #5167 or just print out on plain paper and use as a reference to manually print on tabs in the folder/binder of your choosing.

Binder Tabs: If you would like to preprint binder divider tabs, there are labels set up for use with Avery 8-Tab #11554, Avery 5-Tab #11517, that can be printed on an inkjet printer. There are three files. Each has a different number of tabs which will determine which Avery Tab blanks you will purchase. There are 5-tabs for notebook one, the purple book. There are 8-tabs in notebooks two and three, the white and green notebooks, respectively.

Purchase PDFs, of paperwork and binder labels at gauntletofcaregiving.com.

Organizational Notebook 1:

About our Home Form: This form is the first page in notebook one. This is a two-sided form.

TAB 1: CALENDAR AND SCHEDULE

Calendar: Using the downloadable form or a purchased/punched calendar of choice, it will be placed in the second position for easy access and updating at any time. This is a single-sided form.

TAB 2: DAILY CAREGIVER NOTES

Medication Form: Keep this form updated. Place it first for easy access and reference whenever needed. Using clear tape, paste an example of each pill in line with its description. This is a one-sided form.

Daily Routine Form - this easy to maintain daily record will help to track sleep, activities, diet, eating habits and medication disbursement along with any information of change that should be noted for a physician visit or emergency contact. This is a two-sided form.

TAB 3: IN CASE OF EMERGENCY

Copies Only Coversheet: This cover sheet provides instructions about what documents should have copies included in this section. This is a single-sided form.

In Case of Emergency: This form should be filled out completely. Even though it feels redundant! This is a single-sided form.

Five Wishes Health Directives (Sample): This organization can provide Healthcare directives that meet each State requirements. Refer to Chapter 11 for a more expanded explanation about directives. This is a two-sided form.

TAB 4: POWER OF ATTORNEY

This tab makes it easier to access this important document. It is necessary in order to establish who can do what for a patient's assets and in some states a patient's healthcare.

If a healthcare power of attorney is required, at least a copy of it should be placed here, and other health directives placed in Tab 3. This is a single-sided form.

TAB 5: ESSENTIAL PERSONAL INFORMATION

Essential Personal Information List and Locator List Form - a list of identification, information, and legal documents that need to be created, located, documented, and organized for use when needed. Copies of these items (that are allowed by law) can be included in this section for easy access. A complete list should be included in Notebook 3, Legal and Estate information. This is a two-sided form.

(Note: A copy of the Essential Personal Information Locator list can be added here if the owner is amenable to including it. It is important someone has access to the list. A partial list can be useful for daily access purposes such as WIFI, utility and cable/internet provider company, passwords, etc. The primary list can be kept by the person who is designated as Power of Attorney or conservator, when appropriate. Always seek legal advice before giving anyone access to personal information. Have permission in writing!)

Expense Report Form - This expense report can be downloaded, printed and filled in when appropriate. It is kept in Organizational Notebook #1 so expenses can be filled in daily to keep an accurate account on monies spent on the behalf of whomever is being cared for. It is advisable that all receipts match and accompany any expense report for accurate accountability. This is not an essential form, but an optional form for independently hired or other individually paid caregivers. This is a single-sided form.

Organizational Notebook 2:

TAB 1: PERSONAL HEALTH INFORMATION

Personal Health Information Form - this form provides more in-depth family history and personal health information that is necessary for healthcare visits. This is a two-sided, multi-page form.

TAB 2: HEALTHCARE RECORDS:

Notes Page for Organizational Paperwork Form - this universal form makes it easy and consistent to take notes when in healthcare meetings. URL for download is below in Tab 8. This is a two-sided, multi-page form.

Each time this form is used, it should be included in this section with office visit and discharge summaries. These summaries can be provided in print copies. It is not unusual for them to refer a patient to a portal to download. ASK FOR A PRINT COPY of the office visit summary.

TAB 3: PHYSICIAN INFORMATION:

Physician Information form explanation is found in Chapter 11. There are two forms, primary physician(s) and specialty physician(s). This is a single-sided form.

TAB 4: HOSPITAL INFORMATION:

This form can be used for multiple admissions to a single hospital. Use an additional form for a different hospital. Include discharge paperwork in TAB 2. This is a single-sided form.

TAB 5: VETERANS HEALTH INFORMATION:

This form is filled out for any veteran healthcare. If more than one location is used, fill out a form for each. This is a single-sided form.

TAB 6: NURSING HOME/REHAB INFORMATION:

This form can be used for multiple admissions. Use one form per facility to keep track of records and services. This is a single-sided form.

TAB 7: DME MEDICAL EQUIPMENT:

Important: See Chapter 11 for a full explanation of this form! Knowing how to use it can save money and frustration. This is a single-sided form.

TAB 8: APPOINTMENT NOTE BLANKS:

Blank forms for storage. Print out at least two copies per physician in advance. This is a two-sided form.

Organizational Notebook 3:

SECURITY FIRST - This notebook and the documents it contains should be kept in a secure location or with an Attorney. Usernames and passwords change, so updates should be made on a regular basis as well as all other documents. Update wills, trusts, power of attorney, health directives or other legal documents when anything changes in a person's daily living situation. Also update legal documents at least every five (5) years or if the designated person or entity who created documents is no longer available.

Essential Personal Information Locator List Form - a list of identification, information, and legal documents that have been created, located, documented, and organized for use when needed. Copies of these items (that are allowed by law) can be included in Notebook #1 for easy access. A complete list should reside here and kept in a safe place or with a designated person or entity such as an Attorney's office. This is a two-sided form.

(Note: A copy of the Essential Personal Information Locator list can be added in Notebook #1 if the owner is amenable to including it. It is important someone has access to the list. A partial list can be useful for daily access purposes such as WIFI, utility and cable/internet provider company, passwords, etc. The primary list can be kept by the person who is designated as Power of Attorney or conservator, when appropriate. Always seek legal advice before giving anyone access to personal information. Have permission to access or use on someone else's behalf in writing!)

TAB 1: ATTORNEY-ACCOUNTANT:

Use one sheet for each type of attorney. Examples and definitions of attorney specialties can be found in Chapter 11. "How To Organize Everyday Paperwork." The same for accountant specialties. This is a single-sided form.

TAB 2: POWER OF ATTORNEY

This section is for original documents that are not held by someone else. If documents reside in a specific place notation can be made here and included in the "Important Information" locator list. No form provided.

TAB 3: PERSONAL FINANCIAL:

This section can include bank account paperwork such a check, savings, bonds, stocks, which would be found here or elsewhere and included in the "Essential Personal Information" locator list. No form provided.

TAB 4: ESTATE PLANNING:

To help with estate planning, this document is a glossary of terms that will help to initiate, recognize, and collect what is considered estate documents. A copy or original estate planning documents can be placed here. Any changes, additions, or other information should be included here and or if not, either way, include on the "Important Information" locator list. No form provided.

TAB 5: SECURITY USERNAME & PASSWORDS:

This form is important and should be kept up to date. A copy can be placed elsewhere but is not recommended to be placed in any unsecured location. This is a two-sided form.

TAB 6: FINAL ARRANGEMENTS:

This comprehensive form will help family and loved ones through the difficult decisions needing to be made when loss occurs. It will truly be a blessing to have everything in one place in writing. This is a two-sided, multi-page form.

TAB 7: LAST WILL & TESTAMENT:

This document can be kept here, or notation can be made where it will be held. Also include the location on the "Important Information" locator form. No form provided.

TAB 8: MISCELLANEOUS ORIGINAL DOCUMENTS:

This section is for any legal, financial, or other documents that need to be kept confidential. Items such as original DD214, government records that are not financials such as birth certificate, citizenship records, marriage licenses, death certificates, etc. Also documents that may be important for future financial assistance such as proof of real estate or assets sold.

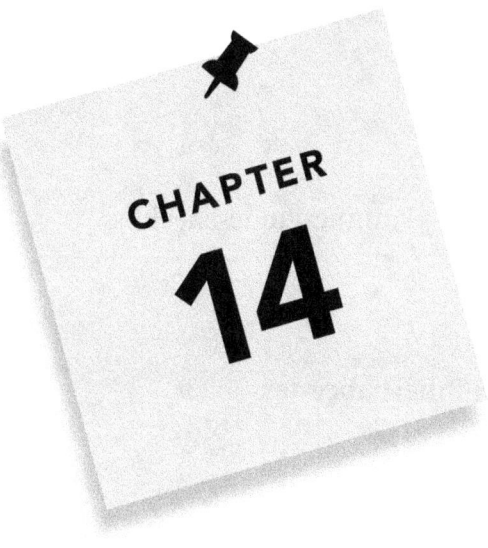

CHAPTER

14

Resources

The resources found on this, and all Resource Pages, will change from time to time depending on State and Government laws and the organizations who provide the services. Revisit these websites regularly to ensure the website link is current for access and so you can be assured you are accessing the most current information.

WARNING: Always double check the website address. There are a lot of fraudulent websites with added extensions or slight changes to addresses who try to mimic businesses and organizations to sell goods or collect personal information and money.

Resources for all Caregiving needs.

Family Caregiver Alliance (FCA)
Based in California
Website: caregiver.org
Find services in your State

Aging with Dignity
Provides guidance for Aging.
Website: agingwithdignity.org

Five Wishes
A program of Aging With Dignity providing Health
Care Directive Guidance and documents in all States
in America except Kansas, New Hampshire, Ohio or
Texas. In these States there may be additional
documents/formats needed.
Website: fivewishes.org

National Council on Aging (NCOA)
Estate Planning Advice and Lawyer Connections Program
Website: https://www.ncoa.org/adviser/estate-planning/estate-planning-guide-checklist/

Tax Foundation
Search Estate Tax by State
Website: taxfoundation.org/data/all/state/state-estate-tax-inheritance-tax-2023/

Resources for self-care as a caregiver.

Wellness
Wellnessinstitute.org
Caregiver.va.gov
Nia.nih.gov

Resources for Medicaid Long Term Care Guidance

Eligibility Requirements by State:
https://www.medicaidplanningassistance.org/state-specific-medicaid-eligibility/

How Medicaid Calculates the Penalty Period for Look-Back Violations
https://www.medicaidplanningassistance.org/penalty-period-divisor/#definition

Child Caregiver Exception
https://www.medicaidplanningassistance.org/child-caregiver-exemption/

Medicaid Planners: Pros & Cons of Public and Private Assistance
https://www.medicaidplanningassistance.org/types-of-medicaid-planners/

Check eligibility:
https://www.medicaidplanningassistance.org/find-a-medicaid-planner/#step=0

APPENDIX

Section One: Acronyms for Healthcare
Section Two: Acronyms: Continuing/Congregate Care Housing and Health Agencies.
Section Three: Medicaid Information by State
Section Four: Samples of Forms for Organizational Paperwork

SECTION ONE

Acronyms for Healthcare

DISCLAIMER: These acronyms have been gathered from many sources and do not represent all healthcare abbreviations which are continually changing. These are for reference only and should not be construed as a medical diagnosis or medical advice. Always consult with a healthcare provider and professional before assuming any definition. Each industry or State may have different acronyms. These represent common or often used and do not constitute a complete and accurate list of all healthcare abbreviations or acronyms.

Acronym	Meaning
A	
A.A.R.O.M.	active assistive range of motion
AAC	augmentative and alternative communication
A.B.G	arterial blood gas
a.c.	before meals
A/C	assist control
ADA Diet	American Diabetes Association Diet
A.D.L.	activities of daily living
A.Fib.	atrial fibrillation
AKA	above-knee amputation or above-the-knee amputation
ALS	amyotrophic lateral sclerosis
AMA	against medical advice
A&O	alert and oriented
A/P	anterior–posterior
A.R.O.M.	active range of motion
ASAP	as soon as possible
ASD	autism spectrum disorder
ASL	American Sign Language
B	
b.i.d.	twice a day
BKA	below-knee amputation

B/L	bilateral
B.L.BS	bilateral breath sounds
BMR	basal metabolism rate
BP	blood pressure
BR	bed rest
bs	bowel sounds
BS	breath sounds
B/S	bedside
bx	biopsy
C	
c̄	with
C	Celsius, centigrade
C1, C2, etc.	first cervical vertebrae, second cervical vertebrae, etc.
CA	cardiac arrest
CA, ca	cancer, carcinoma
CABG	coronary artery bypass graft
CAD	coronary artery disease
cal	calorie
cath	catheter
CBC	complete blood count
cc	cubic centimeter
CC	chief complaint
CHF	congestive heart failure, chronic heart failure
CCU	coronary care unit
CHI	closed head injury
cm	centimeter
CMT	continuing medication and treatment
CN	cranial nerve
CNA	certified nursing assistant
CNS	central nervous system
c/o	complains of
COTA	certified occupational therapy assistant
cont	continue(d)
COPD	chronic obstructive pulmonary disease
CP	cerebral palsy
CPAP	continuous positive airway pressure
CPR	cardiopulmonary resuscitation
CRF	chronic renal failure
CRNP	certified registered nurse practitioner
CSF	cerebrospinal fluid
CT	computerized tomography

CV	cardiovascular
CVA	cerebral vascular accident
CXR	chest X-ray

D

d	day
d/c	discontinue
DC	discharge
DM	diabetes mellitus
DNK	do not know
DNKA	did not keep appointment
DNR	do not resuscitate
DNT	did not test
DOA	dead on arrival
DOB	date of birth
DOE	dyspnea on exertion
d/t	due to
Dx	diagnosis

E

ECC, EKG	electrocardiogram
ED	emergency department
EEG	electroencephalogram
EENT	eyes, ears, nose, throat
EMG	electromyogram
ENT	ears, nose, throat
ER	emergency room
ETOH	ethanol (alcohol)
exam	examination
ext	external, exterior

F

F	Fahrenheit
FH	family history
fib	fibrillation
fl, fld	fluid
FOB	foot of bed
f/u	follow-up
FWB	full weight bearing
Fx	fracture

G

GB	gall bladder
GCS	Glasgow Coma Scale
GE	gastroenterology

GERD	gastroesophageal reflux disease
G/E	gastroenteritis
gen	general
gest.	gestation
G.I.	gastrointestinal
GNA	geriatric nursing assistant
gluc	glucose
GP	general practitioner, general paralysis
GSW	gunshot wound
GTT	glucose tolerance test
Gt. tr.	gait training
GYN	gynecology
H	
h	hour
H/A	headache
HAV	hepatitis A virus
Hb.	hemoglobin
HB	heart block
HBP	high blood pressure
h.d.	at bedtime
HEENT	head, eyes, ears, nose, throat
HEP	home exercise program
H2O	water
h/o	history of
HOB	head of bed
H&P	history and physical
HR	heart rate
HTN	hypertension
HVD	hypertensive vascular disease
Hx	history
Hz	hertz (cycles/second)
I	
ICCU	intensive coronary care unit
ICP	intracranial pressure
ICU	intensive care unit
imp.	impression
incr.	increased(ing)
inf	infusion, inferior
inspire	inspiration, inspiratory
int.	internal
I&O	intake and output

IPPB	intermittent positive pressure breathing
irreg.	irregular
IV	intravenous(ly)
J	
J, jt.	joint
K	
K	potassium, kidney
L	
L	left, liver, liter, lower, light, lumbar
L2, L3	second lumbar vertebrae, third lumbar vertebrae
lab	laboratory
lac.	laceration
lat.	lateral
LBW	low birth rate
L.E.	lower extremities
liq.	liquid
L.O.C.	loss of consciousness, level of consciousness, laxative of choice
LOS	length of stay
LP	lumbar puncture
LPN	licensed practical nurse
LUE	left upper extremity
Lx	larynx
L&W	living and well
M	
m, M	married, male, mother, murmur, meter, mass, molar
max.	maximum, maxillary
MBC	maximum breathing capacity
MBSS	modified barium swallow study
MCA	middle cerebral artery
MD	muscular dystrophy
mdnt.	midnight
med.	medicine
mets.	metastasis
MG	myasthenia gravis
MI	myocardial infarction
min	minute
MICU	medical intensive care unit
mod	moderate
MRI	magnetic resonance imaging
MRSA	methicillin-resistant Staphylococcus aureus
mss	massage

MVA	motor vehicle accident

N

n.	nerve
Na	sodium
NaCl	sodium chloride
NAD	no abnormality detected
NAD	no apparent distress
neg.	negative
neur.	neurology
NG	nasogastric
NIC	neonatal intensive care
NICU	neonatal intensive care unit
NKA	no known allergies
no.	number
NOS	not otherwise specified
NPO	nothing by mouth
NSA	no specific abnormality
NST	nonstress test
N&V	nausea and vomiting
NVD	nausea, vomiting, diarrhea
N&W	normal and well
NWB	non−weight bearing
NYD	not yet diagnosed

O

o	none, without
O	oral
O2	oxygen
O2 cap.	oxygen capacity
O2 sat.	oxygen saturation
OA	osteoarthritis
OB, OBG	obstetrics
OB/GYN	obstetrics and gynecology
Obs	observation
OBS	organic brain syndrome
ODD	oppositional defiant disorder
O/E	on examination
OH	occupational history
OHD	organic heart disease
oint.	ointment
O.M.	otitis media
O.M.E.	otitis media with effusion
OOB, oob	out of bed

Op.	operation
ot.	ear
Oto	otolaryngology
OTC	over-the-counter (pharmaceuticals)
O.T.	occupational therapy, old tuberculin
OR	operating room

P

PA	physician's assistant
p&a	percussion and auscultation
PACU	post anesthesia care unit
PAF	paroxysmal atrial fibrillation
palp.	palpate, palpated, palpable
Path	pathology
PA view	posterior–anterior view on X-ray
p/c, p.c.	after meals
PD	Parkinson's disease
pdr.	powder
PDN	private duty nurse
PE	physical exam, pulmonary embolism, pressure equalizer (tubes)
Ped.	pediatrics
PEEP	positive end-expiratory pressure
PEG	percutaneous endoscopic gastrostomy
PET	positron emission tomography
PH	past history
pharm	pharmacy
PHYS.	physical, physiology
PI	present illness, pulmonary insufficiency
PICU	pulmonary intensive care unit
PID	pelvic inflammatory disease
plts.	platelets
P.M.	afternoon, postmortem
PMH	past medical history
PMR	physical medicine and rehabilitation
PN	poorly nourished, practical nurse
P&N	psychiatry and neurology
PNA	pneumo, pneumonia
PNI	peripheral nerve injury
PNX	pneuomothorax
p.o.	by mouth
p.o.d.	postoperative day
pos.	positive

post.	posterior
POSTOP.	postoperative
pot. or potass.	potassium
PR	proctology
pre-op	preoperative
prep.	prepare for
p.r.m.	according to circumstances
p.r.n., PRN	as often as necessary, as needed
prod.	productive
Prog.	prognosis
PROM	passive range of motion
pron.	pronator, pronation
prosth.	prosthesis
PSH	past surgical history
Psych.	psychiatry
pt., Pt.	patient
PT, P.T.	physical therapy
PTA	prior to admission
PTA pulse	posterior tibial artery pulse
PUD	peptic ulcer disease
PVD	peripheral vascular disease
PVT	previous trouble
PWB%	partial weight bearing with percent
Px, PX	physical examination

Q

q	every
q.h.	every hour
q.i.d.	four times a day
qt.	quart
quad.	quadriplegic

R

R, r	right
R.	rub, rectal temperature
RA	rheumatoid arthritis, right atrium
rad.	radial
r.a.m.	rapid alternating movements
R.A.S.	right arm sitting
RAtx	radiation therapy
rbc/RBC	red blood cell, red blood count
RCA	right coronary artery
RCU	respiratory care unit

RD	respiratory distress
RDS	respiratory distress syndrome
RE	reconditioning exercise
reg.	regular
rehab.	rehabilitation
resp.	respiratory, respirations
RF	rheumatic fever
RLAS	Rancho Los Amigos Scale
R to L&A	react to light and accommodation
RLE	right lower extremity
RN	registered nurse
RND	radical neck dissection
RO, R/O	rule out
ROM	range of motion, rupture of membranes, right otitis media
ROS	review of symptoms
Rt.	right
RT	radiation therapy, respiratory therapy
RUE	right upper extremity
RV	residual volume
RW	rolling walker
Rx	therapy, prescription
S	
s	without
S	sensation, sensitive, serum
Sa.	saline
s.c.	subcutaneous(ly)
Scc	squamous cell carcinoma
SCCA	squamous cell carcinoma, squamous cell carcinoma antigen
SCD	sudden cardiac death
SCI	spinal cord injury
schiz	schizophrenia
SCU	special care unit
sec	second
Sens.	sensory, sensation
sep.	separated
SGA	small for gestational age
s.gl.	without correction (without glasses)
SH	social history
SI	stroke index
sib.	sibling
SICU	surgical intensive care unit

SIDS	sudden infant death syndrome
skel.	skeletal
Sl.	slightly
SL	under the tongue
SLP	speech-language pathologist
sm	small
SNF	skilled nursing facility
SOAP	subjective, objective, assessment, plan
SOB	shortness of breath
S/P, s/p	status post (previous condition)
sp. cd.	spinal cord
spec.	specimen
sp. fl.	spinal fluid
sp&H	speech and hearing
spin.	spine, spinal
spont.	spontaneous
s/s	signs and symptoms
SS	social service
ST	speech therapy
stat., STAT	immediately
STD	sexually transmitted disease
subcut.	subcutaneous
subling.	sublingual
sup.	superior
supin.	supination
surg.	surgery, surgical
Sx	symptoms
sys.	system
Syst.	systolic
Sz	seizure
T	
T	temperature
T&A	tonsils and adenoids, tonsillectomy and adenoidectomy
tab.	tablet
TAH	total abdominal hysterectomy
TB	tuberculosis
TBI	traumatic brain injury
temp	temperature
THERAP.	therapy, therapeutic
THR	total hip replacement
TIA	transient ischemic attack

TKR	total knee replacement
TNM	tumor, nodes, and metastases
TO	telephone order
TPN	total parenteral nutrition
TPR	temperature, pulse, respiration
tr	trace
trach	tracheostomy
tsp.	teaspoon
Tx	treatment, traction
U	
U/A	urinalysis
UCD, UCHD	usual childhood diseases
UG	upward gaze
Unilat.	unilateral
u/o	under observation
Ur.	urine
URD	upper respiratory disease
URI	upper respiratory infection
Urol.	urology
u/s, US	ultrasound
UTI	urinary tract infection
V	
V	vein
VA	visual acuity
vag	vagina, vaginal
VC, vit.cap.	vital capacity
VD	venereal disease
vent.	ventilator
vert.	vertical
VF	visual fields, ventricular fibrillation
VFSS	videofluoroscopic swallowing study
Via	by way of
vit.	vitamin
VN	visiting nurse
VO	verbal order
VS, V.S.	vital signs
W	
w, wk	week
W/C, wh.ch.	wheelchair
WBT	weight bearing tolerance
WFL	within functional limits

w/n	within
WNL	within normal limits
WP	whirlpool
wt.	weight
w/u	workup
X	
x	times
Y	
y.o.	years old
yrs.	years

SECTION TWO

Acronyms: Continuing/Congregate Care Housing and Health Agencies

For more acronyms https://aspe.hhs.gov/common-acronyms

Acronym	Agency Description	Category	Website-Reference
ACL	Administration for Community Living	ACL	acl.gov
ACL	Aging and Disability Resources Centers	ACL	acl.gov
ASPE	Adult Family/Foster Care Home	ALF	aspe.hhs.gov
AHC	Agency for Health Care Administration		ahcancal.org
ALF	Assisted Living Facility	ALF	Use local search
ACL	Administration on Aging	ACL	acl.gov
ACL	Association of Programs for Rural Independent Living	ACL	acl.gov
NIA NIH	Continuing Care Retirement Communities	LCC	nia.nih.gov
	Caregiver/Caretaker		Use local search
ACL	Disability Information and Access Line	ACL	acl.gov
ECC	Extended Congregate Care	ALF	aspe.hhs.gov
FOIA	Freedom of Information Act	ACL	acl.gov
HHS	Home Health Services		Use local search
LCC	Life Care Communities	ACL	nia.nih.gov
LMH	Limited Mental Health services	ALF	aspe.hhs.gov
LNS	Limited Nursing Services	ALF	aspe.hhs.gov
NCAL	National Center for Assisted Living		ahcancal.org
NCIL	National Council on Independent Living	ACL	acl.gov
NDRN	National Disabilities Rights Network	ACL	acl.gov
NFCS	National Family Caregiver Services	ACL	acl.gov
OAA	Older Americans Act	ACL	acl.gov
OSS	Optional State Supplement	ALF	aspe.hhs.gov

SECTION THREE

State	Phone Number	Website
Alaska	(800) 780-9972	https://health.alaska.gov/dpa/Pages/medicaid/default.aspx
Alabama	(800) 362-1504	https://medicaid.alabama.gov/
Arkansas	(800) 457-4454	https://humanservices.arkansas.gov/
Arizona	(855)-HEA-PLUS	https://www.azahcccs.gov/AHCCCS/AboutUs/programdescription.html
California	(800) 541-5555	https://www.dhcs.ca.gov/services
Colorado	(800) 221-3943	https://www.healthfirstcolorado.com/
Connecticut	(800) 842-2159	https://portal.ct.gov/OHA/Health-Care-Plans/Other-Plans/Medicaid
Washington DC	(202) 727-5355	https://dhcf.dc.gov/service/medicaid
Delaware	(866) 843-7212	https://dhss.delaware.gov/dmma/
Florida	(866) 762-2237	https://www.benefits.gov/benefit/1625
Georgia	(877) 423-4746	https://medicaid.georgia.gov/
Hawaii	(800) 316-8005	https://medquest.hawaii.gov/
Iowa	(800) 338-8366	https://hhs.iowa.gov/programs/welcome-iowa-medicaid
Idaho	(877) 456-1233	https://healthandwelfare.idaho.gov/services-programs/medicaid-health
Illinois	(800) 843-6154	https://www.benefits.gov/benefit/1628
Indiana	(800) 403-0864	https://www.in.gov/medicaid/
Kansas	(800) 792-4884	https://kancare.ks.gov/
Kentucky	(855) 306-8959	https://www.chfs.ky.gov/agencies/dms/Pages/default.aspx
Massachusetts	(800) 841-2900	https://www.mass.gov/topics/masshealth
Michigan	(855) 789-5610	https://www.michigan.gov/mdhhs/assistance-programs/medicaid
Minnesota	(800) 657-3739	https://mn.gov/dhs/people-we-serve/adults/health-care/health-care-programs/programs-and-services/medical-assistance.jsp
Missouri	(855) 373-9994	https://mydss.mo.gov/healthcare

Mississippi	(800) 421-2408	https://medicaid.ms.gov/
Montana	(888) 706-1535	https://dphhs.mt.gov/montanahealthcareprograms/memberservices
North Carolina	(877) 201-3750	https://medicaid.ncdhhs.gov/
North Dakota	(800) 472-2622	https://www.hhs.nd.gov/healthcare/medicaid
Nebraska	(855) 632-7633	https://dhhs.ne.gov/Pages/medicaid-and-long-term-care.aspx
New Hampshire	(844) ASK-DHHS	https://www.dhhs.nh.gov/programs-services/medicaid
New Jersey	(800) 701-0710	https://www.nj.gov/humanservices/dmahs/clients/medicaid/
New Mexico	(800) 283-4465	https://nmmedicaid.portal.conduent.com/static/index.htm
Nevada	(877) 638-3472	https://www.medicaid.nv.gov/
New York	(800) 541-2831	https://www.health.ny.gov/health_care/medicaid/
Ohio	(800) 324-8680	https://medicaid.ohio.gov/
Oklahoma	(800) 987-7767	https://oklahoma.gov/ohca.html
Rhode Island	(855) 840-4774	https://healthsourceri.com/medicaid/
South Carolina	(888) 549-0820	https://www.scdhhs.gov/
South Dakota	(605) 773-4678	https://dss.sd.gov/medicaid/
Tennessee	(855) 259-0701	https://www.tn.gov/tenncare/members-applicants/eligibility/tenncare-medicaid.html
Texas	(800) 252-9240	https://www.hhs.texas.gov/services/health/medicaid-chip
Utah	(866) 435-7414	https://medicaid.utah.gov/
Virginia	(800) 643-2273	https://www.dmas.virginia.gov/
Vermont	(800) 250-8427	http://dvha.vermont.gov/members
Washington	(877) 501-2233	https://www.dshs.wa.gov/altsa/home-and-community-services/medicaid
Wisconsin	(800) 947-3529	https://www.dhs.wisconsin.gov/medicaid/index.htm
West Virginia	(800) 318-2956	https://dhhr.wv.gov/bms/Pages/default.aspx
Wyoming	(307) 777-7531	https://health.wyo.gov/healthcarefin/medicaid/

SECTION FOUR

Organizational Notebook Pages

The companion pages can be purchased online from the resource where you purchased this book. The pages and tabs in the packet to be used in your own choice of notebooks or purchase suggested notebooks in Chapter 12, Binders and Such. In the future these notebooks may be purchased already set up, ready to fill out and go anywhere. Return to the resource where you purchased this book or go to gauntletofcaregiving.com

~Daily Caregiving~

Checklist for Calendar & Schedule section in order:

- ☐ About Us & Our Home Form (First Page before Divider)
- ☐ Calendar/Schedule (After Divider)

Organizational Notebook #1
"Purple"

Belongs To:

_____

The Gauntlet of Caregiving

About US

Name _____

Our Address		Nearest Cross Street
Land Line/Cell Phone		
	IN CASE OF EMERGENCY	CALL 911

OUR FRIENDS, FAMILY and PETS

FRIENDS AND NEIGHBORS

☐
☐
☐
☐
☐
☐

FAMILY - GO TO IN CASE OF EMERGENCY SHEET

☐
☐
☐
☐
☐
☐

PET(S)/LIVESTOCK/OTHER

☐
☐
☐
☐
☐
☐

OTHER INFORMATION - NOTIFY FOR SCHEDULE CHANGES

CARE GIVING SERVICES	SCHEDULE	CONTACT	ACTIVE YES/NO

UTILITIES	ACCOUNT #	PASSWORD	NAME ON ACCT

IN CASE OF EMERGENCY: THIS BOOK (PURPLE) AND THE HEALTH INFORMATION BOOK (WHITE) CONTAIN INFORMATION ABOUT THE PATIENT!

METHOD OF CONTACT AND OTHER DETAILS	CONTACT NAME	ADDITIONAL INFORMATION

MONTH _____

YEAR _____

CALENDAR NAME _____

SUNDAY	MONDAY	TUESDAY	WEDNESDAY	THURSDAY	FRIDAY	SATURDAY

MONTH _____

YEAR _____

CALENDAR NAME _____

SUNDAY	MONDAY	TUESDAY	WEDNESDAY	THURSDAY	FRIDAY	SATURDAY

Weekly schedule

Week of: _____

DATE: _____

	SUNDAY	MONDAY	TUESDAY	WEDNESDAY	THURSDAY	FRIDAY	SATURDAY
8:00 AM							
8:30 AM							
9:00 AM							
9:30 AM							
10:00 AM							
10:30 AM							
11:00 AM							
11:30 AM							
12:00 PM							
12:30 PM							
1:00 PM							
1:30 PM							
2:00 PM							

	SUNDAY	MONDAY	TUESDAY	WEDNESDAY	THURSDAY	FRIDAY	SATURDAY
2:30 PM							
3:00 PM							
3:30 PM							
4:00 PM							
4:30 PM							
5:00 PM							
5:30 PM							
6:00 PM							
6:30 PM							
7:00 PM							
7:30 PM							
8:00 PM							
8:30 PM							
9:00 PM							
9:30 PM							
10:00 PM							
10:30 PM							
11:00 PM							

~Daily Caregiving~

Checklist for Daily Caregiver Notes section in order:

☐ Medication List

☐ Daily Caregiving Notes Filled Out (Most recent date first)

Organizational Notebook #1

"Purple"

DAILY ROUTINE

1|2|3|4|5|6|7|8|9|10|11|12|13|14|15|16|17|18|19|20|21|22|23|24|25|26|27|28|29|30|31

January | February | March | April | May | June | July | August | September | October | November | December

Monday | Tuesday | Wednesday | Thursday | Friday |Saturday | Sunday

--ONE SHEET PER DAY ----------------------------------

CARE GIVER: _____   Day Normal: Y   N   If N, Reason: _____

MEAL: Breakfast   Lunch   Snack   Dinner/Supper   Snack   Time: _____ AM / PM

Daily notes: _____

_____

_____

_____

CARE GIVER: _____   Day Normal: Y   N   If N, Reason: _____

MEAL: Breakfast   Lunch   Snack   Dinner/Supper   Snack   Time: _____ AM / PM

Daily notes: _____

_____

_____

_____

CARE GIVER: _____   Day Normal: Y   N   If N, Reason: _____

MEAL: Breakfast   Lunch   Snack   Dinner/Supper   Snack   Time: _____ AM / PM

Daily notes: _____

_____

_____

_____

Page _____ of _____   Via: Phone | Meeting |Other _____

CARE GIVER: _____ Day Normal: Y N   If N, Reason: _____

MEAL: Breakfast Lunch Snack Dinner/Supper Snack Time: _____ AM / PM

Daily notes: _____

_____

_____

_____

_____

CARE GIVER: _____ Day Normal: Y N   If N, Reason: _____

MEAL: Breakfast Lunch Snack Dinner/Supper Snack Time: _____ AM / PM

Daily notes: _____

_____

_____

_____

_____

Activities(Exercise/PT/OT) & Hygiene Care (Bathing/Sponge Bath/Other such as Wound Care)

_____

_____

_____

_____

_____

_____

_____

_____

_____

Page _____ of _____   Via: Phone | Meeting |Other _____

~Daily Caregiving~

Checklist for In Case of Emergency section in order:

- ☐ In Case of Emergency (ICE) Information Sheet
- ☐ Personal Information Sheet
- ☐ Healthcare Directive (Copies)

Organizational Notebook #1
"Purple"

The Gauntlet of Caregiving

In Case of Emergency (ICE)

This is a list of what to do and who to contact when an emergency happens.

It will be helpful for either you or someone else to more efficiently take care of the situation.

If Emergency happens at <u>HOME</u>:

1. Contact EMS   FIRST! _____ Phone: _____
2. Contact EMS (Other) _____ Phone: _____
3. Contact Family/Friend _____ Phone: _____
4. Contact Family/Friend _____ Phone: _____
5. Contact Caregiver Employer _____ Phone: _____
6. Locate DNR & Health Care Directives or
   Healthcare Surrogate _____ Phone: _____

If Emergency happens at an <u>INDEPENDENT LIVING OR ASSISTED LIVING</u> facility:

1. Contact EMS   FIRST! _____ Phone: _____
2. Contact EMS (Other) _____ Phone: _____
3. Contact Front Desk_____ Phone: _____
4. Contact Family/Friend _____ Phone: _____
5. Contact Family/Friend _____ Phone: _____
6. Contact Caregiver Employer _____ Phone: _____
7. Locate DNR & Health Care Directives or
   Healthcare Surrogate _____ Phone: _____

- o **<u>Include: Copy of Health Care Directives in this section.</u>**

<u>IMPORTANAT NOTE:</u> *If a Healthcare Directive or Health Surrogate <u>is not notified, a DNR</u> could take precedence in an emergency care situation. Talk to your Attorney or Healthcare provider to make sure all healthcare directives fulfill your wishes and do not conflict.*

Example: The patient may not want to be on life support or not want excessive resuscitation, but may want the use of a defibrillator for resuscitation.

COPIES

ONLY

~

POWER OF
ATTORNEY

~

HEALTH CARE
DIRECTIVES

~

DNR

~

COPIES

ONLY

The Gauntlet of Caregiving

FIVE WISHES®

MY WISH FOR:

The Person I Want to Make Care Decisions for Me When I Can't
1

The Kind of Medical Treatment I Want or Don't Want
2

How Comfortable I Want to Be
3

How I Want People to Treat Me
4

What I Want My Loved Ones to Know
5

_____

Print Your Name

_____

Birthdate

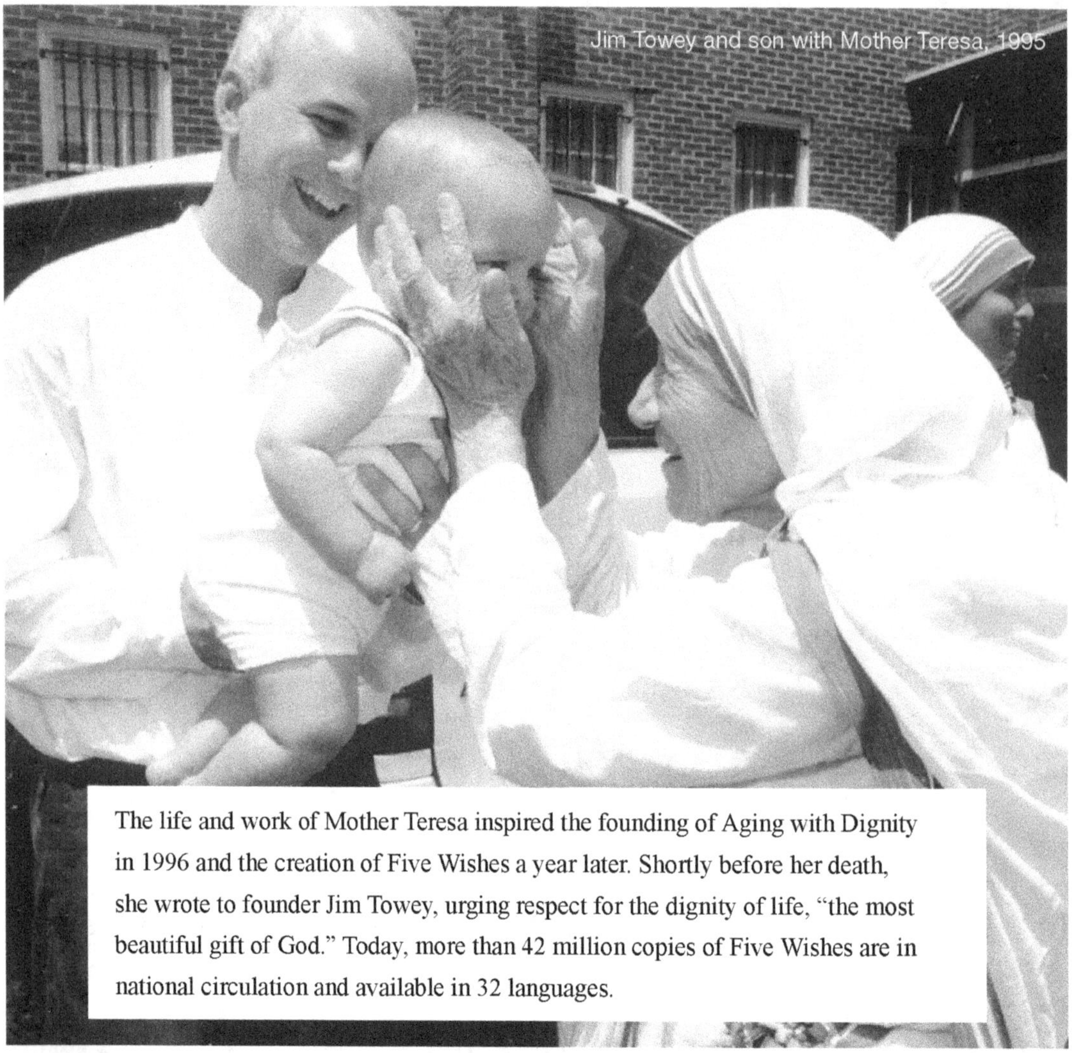

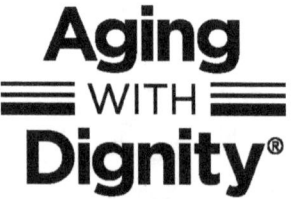

Jim Towey and son with Mother Teresa, 1995

The life and work of Mother Teresa inspired the founding of Aging with Dignity in 1996 and the creation of Five Wishes a year later. Shortly before her death, she wrote to founder Jim Towey, urging respect for the dignity of life, "the most beautiful gift of God." Today, more than 42 million copies of Five Wishes are in national circulation and available in 32 languages.

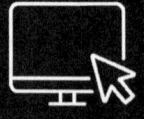

Check out more information on advance care planning at *FiveWishes.org/resources*

To order or for any questions about Five Wishes:

(888) 5-WISHES or (888) 594-7437

www.FiveWishes.org

Five Wishes is a program of:

Aging WITH Dignity®

P.O. Box 1661
Tallahassee, Florida 32302

 Aging with Dignity wishes to thank Oregon Health Decisions for contributing to the drafting of wish number two, and Kate Callahan, Charles Sabatino, and Tere Saenz for their help.

~Daily Caregiving~

Checklist for Power of Attorney & DNR section:

☐ DNR – Do Not Resuscitate (Copy)

☐ Power of Attorney (Copy)

Organizational Notebook #1
"Purple"

POWER OF ATTORNEY

The Gauntlet of Caregiving

~Daily Caregiving~

Checklist for Important Personal Information List section:

- ☐ Important Personal Information Checklist
- ☐ Important Personal Information Locator List (Limited or Optional)

Organizational Notebook #1
"Purple"

The Gauntlet of Caregiving

IMPORTANT PERSONAL INFORMATION LIST

This information and its location should be readily available to the person who will be a caregiver if ever needed. Whether a Spouse, Child, Relative or Friend/Guardian, it is imperative that someone has access so that YOU can be taken care of when needed.

If there is a confidence or conflict issue, a third party such as an Attorney or Guardian should be assigned to hold this information.

Gather this information, then place in the recommended three "Organizational Notebooks" recommended in the article "How to organize everyday paperwork – Part 2"

Identification requirements*

- Driver's License(s) or State Issued ID
- Social Security Card(s)
- Birth Certificate
- Proof of Citizenship or Green card
- Passport
- Veteran: DD214 and VA ID "Healthcare Enrollee" card
- Pension Identification Card(s)

Personal Health Information*

- Medicare Card(s)
- Supplemental Health Insurance Cards (Copy front & back)
- Long Term Health Care Insurance
- Dental & Vision Insurance
- Other Health Plans such as VA, Government Employee, or Pension Plans (Do not copy Government ID's especially Military ID's, it is a violation and illegal)
- List of Current Medications, Prescribing Doctor, Use & Dosage (Health History Form)
- List of Current Doctors or Specialty Care Physician(s) (Health History Form)
- List of Doctors Recently Scene in Hospital (Health History Form)
- Health History (Health History Form)
- Living Will (See *Links to State Requirements*)
- Healthcare Directive (See *Links to State Requirements*)
- Healthcare Surrogate Designation (See *Links to State Requirements*)
- Healthcare Power of Attorney (See *Links to State Requirements*)
- DNR – Original signed Do Not Resuscitate form.

The Gauntlet of Caregiving – A Guide For Non-Professionals Who Give Care To Family and Friends
Gauntlet of Caregiving – Organizational Notebook 1

Gauntlet of Caregiving   Copyright 2024

Personal Assets and Financial Management*

- o Motor Vehicle Registration or Title (Cars, Campers, Motorcycle, Mobile Homes) If financed, Financial Institution information, copy of loan(s) & Payment Information
- o Income Verification from ALL sources including Pension Benefits
- o Checking/Savings, Brokerage accounts, Statements of all for past 3-6 months
- o Income Tax Filing for last 5 yrs.
- o Mortgage Information (Asset Liability Form)
- o Property Tax Bill(s) & Addresses (The property address does not always appear on the bill)
- o Property Insurance Providers (Homeowners, Vehicle, Boat, Camper, Golf Cart, Motorcycle, etc.)
- o Personal Residence and Value (Required for Government programs that are based on assets and income such as Medicaid, County/City in Home Care, & other programs)
- o Technology Usernames and Passwords for online accounts.
- o Power of Attorney (Durable and/or stated powers)

Legal and Professional*

- o Long-Term Care Insurance Policies
- o Business Papers: Partnership Agreements, Financial Statements, Buy/Sell Agreements
- o Life Insurance and Annuity Policies including current values
- o Funeral Planning Declaration (Include all Details)
- o Trust Agreements or TOD – Transfer on Death Deed for Real Estate
- o Last Will and Testament (Attorney Name or Where is it held)
- o Estate Planning and/or Elder Care Attorney Name and Contact Information

* Gather this information, then place in the recommended three "Organizational Notebooks" instructed in the article "How to organize everyday paperwork – Part 1,2,& 3"

~Healthcare~

Checklist for Personal Health Info. section:

☐ Medication List

☐ Personal Health Information and History Form
Filled In Completely

Organizational Notebook #2
"White"

Belongs To:

_____

MEDICATION LIST FOR _____

Date of Last Update: _____

Name of Medication Medication Name on Bottle	Strength of Medication	Description or Sample	Dosage Instructions	Special Instructions for Dosage	What is this medication for?	Who prescribed? Who filled?	Last Refill Date & Quantity
	10 MG Tab	Tape Sample Here	1/2 Tablet by mouth	A.M. & P.M. on empty stomach	Diagnosis: Heart, A-Fib	Dr. Know Cleveland Clinic	2/2/22 100 pills

MEDICATION LIST FOR _____

Date of Last Update: _____

Name of Medication	Strength of Medication	Description or Sample	Dosage Instructions	Special Instructions for Dosage	What is this medication for?	Who prescribed? Who filled?	Last Refill Date & Quantity
Medication Name on Bottle	10 MG Tab	Tape Sample Here	1/2 Tablet by mouth	A.M. & P.M. on empty stomach	Diagnosis: Heart, A-Fib	Dr. Know Cleveland Clinic	2/2/22 100 pills

Personal Information

Legal Name: First _____ Middle _____ Last _____

Married Name: First _____ Middle _____ Last _____

Birth Name: First _____ Middle _____ Last _____

Birth Date: _____ USA Citizen: Y   N   Military Veteran: Y N Branch: _____

Birth State: _____ Country: _____ Province _____

Current Home Address: _____ City/State/Zip: _____

Primary Address: Y N (If no, provide additional information)

Primary Home Address: _____ City/State/Zip: _____

Emergency Contact Information:

Name: _____ Address: _____

Phone: _____ Relation: _____ Email: _____

Name: _____ Address: _____

Phone: _____ Relation: _____ Email: _____

Name: _____ Address: _____

Phone: _____ Relation: _____ Email: _____

Name: _____ Address: _____

Phone: _____ Relation: _____ Email: _____

Name: _____ Address: _____

Phone: _____ Relation: _____ Email: _____

Personal Preferred method of contact:

__ Email address: _____

__ Phone: Cell: _____ Office: _____ Home: _____

__ Do you wish to have a message left when a call is made? Y N

__ Caregiver or Other: Name: _____/Agency _____

This person's information must be included in the "Emergency Contact Information" with a valid phone number.

Personal Health Information

Medical Insurance:

Insurance Provider: _____ Policy Number: _____

Supplement 1: _____ Policy Number: _____

Supplement 2: _____ Policy Number: _____

Veteran Clinic: _____ Policy Number: _____

Additional: _____ Policy Number: _____

Preferred Pharmacy: _____ Phone Number: _____

Pharmacy Address: _____

Co-Pay: $_____ Per Visit Deductible: $_____ Fulfilled Y N N/A

Are you a member of a Group Plan through a Government Pension? Y N

Hospital Records *for last 2 years. If information is older than 2 years, include dates month/year of admissions. Also include specialty facilities such as University Hospitals, Cancer Treatment Centers, etc.*

Hospital address: _____ City/State/Zip: _____

Reason for admission: _____

Attending physician: _____ Phone:_____

Discharge notes are available: Y N   Dates: _____

Hospital address: _____ City/State/Zip: _____

Reason for admission: _____

Attending physician: _____ Phone:_____

Discharge notes are available: Y N   Dates: _____

Hospital address: _____ City/State/Zip: _____

Reason for admission: _____

Attending physician: _____ Phone:_____

Discharge notes are available: Y N   Dates: _____

Hospital address: _____ City/State/Zip: _____

Reason for admission: _____

Attending physician: _____ Phone:_____

Discharge notes are available: Y N   Dates: _____

Hospital address: _____ City/State/Zip: _____

Reason for admission: _____

Attending physician: _____ Phone:_____

Discharge notes are available: Y N   Dates: _____

Hospital address: _____ City/State/Zip: _____

Reason for admission: _____

Attending physician: _____ Phone:_____

Discharge notes are available: Y N Dates: _____

Hospital address: _____ City/State/Zip: _____

Reason for admission: _____

Attending physician: _____ Phone:_____

Discharge notes are available: Y N Dates: _____

Surgeries Other (MOHS, Cosmetic procedures, etc):

_____   _____   _____

_____   _____   _____

_____   _____   _____

The following information will change continually and will need to be updated for each visit to a doctor or medical facility:

     Have you traveled overseas in the last 6 months? Y N

     Have you been exposed to anyone who is ill within the last 2 weeks? Y N

     Have you fallen within the last 2 weeks prior to the current doctor's visit? Y N

         If yes, what occurred? _____

Vaccine Information:

Did you have the COVID 19 Vaccine? Y N   If yes:__ single shot   __ 2-shot __ Booster 1 2 3

      Name of Vaccine Manufacturer: _____

      Have you had COVID 19? Y N When? _____

      What treatment did you receive? _____

      _____

      Any continuing issues? Y N Describe: _____

Other Vaccines/Date of Vaccine: _____

Other Vaccines/Date of Vaccine: _____

Other Vaccines/Date of Vaccine: _____

Other Vaccines/Date of Vaccine: _____

Other Vaccines/Date of Vaccine: _____

Other vaccines would include Anthrax, Cholera, Diphtheria, Hepatitis A-B, Influenza, Seasonal Flu, Measles, Meningococcal, Mumps, Pertussis, Pneumococcal, Poli, Rabies, Rotavirus, Rubella, Shingles, Smallpox, Tetanus, Tuberculosis, Typhoid Fever, Varicella, Yellow Fever. If these were administered during Military Service, make note of Service dates (example 1950-1954)since vaccines are administered as needed for deployments.

Medication or Vaccine Allergies

Name of Medication/Vaccine: _____ Reaction: _____

      Remedy: _____

Name of Medication/Vaccine: _____ Reaction: _____

      Remedy: _____

Name of Medication/Vaccine: _____ Reaction: _____

      Remedy: _____

Name of Medication/Vaccine: _____ Reaction: _____

      Remedy: _____

Name of Medication/Vaccine: _____ Reaction: _____

      Remedy: _____

Name of Medication/Vaccine: _____ Reaction: _____

      Remedy: _____

Surgeries/Implants

Have you had surgery to remove an organ or add an implant?

Surgery (Removal/Implant) _____

Location where Surgery was done/When: _____

Reason/Diagnosis: _____

Surgery (Removal/Implant) _____

Location where Surgery was done/When: _____

Reason/Diagnosis: _____

Surgery (Removal/Implant) _____

Location where Surgery was done/When: _____

Reason/Diagnosis: _____

Surgery (Removal/Implant) _____

Location where Surgery was done/When: _____

Reason/Diagnosis: _____

Living situation

Do you have a spouse, significant other, partner, child or friend who lives with you? Y N

        If yes, is this person included in your emergency contacts? Y N

Do you have a religious preference? Y N If yes, please describe: _____

Are you a member of an organization such as AARP or AMAC or AAA? Y N   _____

        If yes, please provide information under supplemental health insurance.

Are you a member of a Health Screening program? Y N _____

        If yes, can you provide results of any Health Screening exams you have? Y N

Social Connections

Where did you attend High School?_____

Are you connected with Alumni? Y N If yes, in what way? _____

Where did you attend University/College? _____

Are you connected with Alumni? Y N If yes, in what way? _____

What was your career? _____

Did you have more than one? Y N If yes, describe: _____

Do you stay in touch with co-workers? Y N If yes, in what way? _____

Do you have hobbies or activities you have done in the past? Y N

Describe: _____

Do you have hobbies or activities you do now? Y N Describe: _____

_____

Do you attend a gym, YMCA, or organized exercise activity? Y N

If yes, when, where & how often? _____

Do you attend a Church? Y N If Yes, when, where & how often? _____

If yes, is there anyone that should be contacted? _____

Are you a member of any other community organizations? Y N

If yes, add name, contact, or any other information that is important: _____

Additional Personal Health History Information

This information is often helpful to know when visiting a new physician and may be asked on the initial pre-visit information form.

Are your parents alive? Y N If yes, what are their ages?   Mother:_____ Father _____

Other family members such as Sister(s), Brother(s) alive? Y N If yes, what are their ages?

_____

_____

_____

Be sure to fill out questions about family history completely---

Health questions asked about parents:

High Cholesterol:	__ Father	__ Mother	Result: _____
High blood Pressure	__ Father	__ Mother	Result: _____
Cancer	__ Father	__ Mother	Result: _____
Heart disease	__ Father	__ Mother	Result: _____
Diabetes	__ Father	__ Mother	Result: _____
Dementia	__ Father	__ Mother	Result: _____
Parkinson's disease	__ Father	__ Mother	Result: _____
Thyroid	__ Father	__ Mother	Result: _____
Smoker _____	__ Father	__ Mother	Result: _____
Other_____	__ Father	__ Mother	Result: _____
Other _____	__ Father	__ Mother	Result: _____

Mental health conditions such as:

- alcoholism   __ Father   __ Mother   __ Child   __ Sibling
- depression: __ Father   __ Mother   __ Child   __ Sibling
- PTSD   __ Father   __ Mother   __ Child   __ Sibling
- Other _____   __ Father   __ Mother   __ Child   __ Sibling
- Other _____   __ Father   __ Mother   __ Child   __ Sibling

Have you or anyone you are related to been exposed to water contamination, chemical spills, side stream smoke, or other contaminants? Explain:

_____

_____

_____

_____

_____

_____

_____

_____

Is this exposure connected with Military Service? Y   N

As a result, have you been diagnosed with a disability that has not been mentioned before in this health care information? Y N   If yes, explain:

_____

_____

_____

_____

_____

_____

Additional Information:

_____

_____

_____

_____

_____

Veterans Service Information:

Do you have a DD214? Y N   Can you provide a copy of this document? Y N

Do you have medical records with the VA? Y N If Yes: Are these records available? Y N

If VA records are available, will you provide them? Y N   If no, please provide contact information of the facility where records are located: _____

> NOTE: Important, keep copies of VA facilities and medical facilities in the "Hospital Records" using a "Hospital" cover sheet to separate. Label as" Veteran Facility" in chronological order, most recent first. Veterans Administration information should be separated under "Veterans Administration" and will include official records of service only.

Were you involved in any Conflicts? Y N If more than one, please state all and jobs you performed:

Conflict: _____ Duration of service: _____ # Tours _____
Any disabilities contributed to this service? Y N Describe diagnosis: _____

Conflict: _____ Duration of service: _____ # Tours _____
Any disabilities contributed to this service? Y N Describe diagnosis: _____

Conflict: _____ Duration of service: _____ # Tours _____
Any disabilities contributed to this service? Y N Describe diagnosis: _____

Conflict: _____ Duration of service: _____ # Tours _____
Do you have disabilities contributed to this service? Y N Describe diagnosis including percentage of disability if not included in health information: _____

_____

_____

_____

As a Veteran or Spouse of a Veteran, do you receive Aid & Attendance? Y N   If yes, please describe:

_____

_____

Additional Information:

~Healthcare~

Checklist for Healthcare Records section:

☐ Healthcare Records In chronological order, most recent first.

☐ Use Appointment Notes for office visits and include with visit summary.

Take this book and Notebook #1 with "Daily Routine" notes to every Physician visit for reference.

Organizational Notebook #2
"White"

The Gauntlet of Caregiving

The Gauntlet of Caregiving – HEALTHCARE - Organizational Notebook 2
These Note Forms move to "Healthcare Records" accompanied by a Summary of Office/Hospital Visit filed in
Chronological Order keeping the most recent information on top for easy access.

1|2|3|4|5|6|7|8|9|10|11|12|13|14|15|16|17|18|19|20|21|22|23|24|25|26|27|28|29|30|31

January | February | March | April | May | June | July | August | September | October | November | December

Monday | Tuesday | Wednesday | Thursday | Friday |Saturday | Sunday

Time: _____ AM | PM

Provider of Service _____ Location _____

Future Appointments: _____ ○ Same location or ○ Different location

Location if different: _____

Concerns, Diagnosis, Plan and Notes from this appointment:

_____

_____

_____

_____

_____

_____

_____

_____

_____

_____

_____

_____

_____

_____

_____

_____

_____

Page _____ of _____   Via: Phone | Meeting |Other _____

These Note Forms move to "Healthcare Records" accompanied by a Summary of Office/Hospital Visit filed in
Chronological Order keeping the most recent information on top for easy access.

Continued

_____

_____

_____

_____

_____

_____

_____

_____

_____

_____

_____

_____

_____

_____

_____

_____

_____

_____

_____

_____

_____

_____

Page _____ of _____   Via: Phone | Meeting |Other _____

~Healthcare~

Checklist for Physician Information section:

☐ Physician Information sheet

-Primary Physician(s) sometimes there will be a VA primary and an Insurance primary

☐ Specialty Physician Information sheet

-These would be Physicians who specialize in a specific field such a Pulmonary, Cardiology, Vascular, Vision, Oncology, etc.

Organizational Notebook #2
"White"

The Gauntlet of Caregiving

Physician Name: _____

Office Name: _____

Phone Number: _____

Address: _____

Associated facility:

- o Primary Care: _____

- o Hospital: _____

- o Cancer Center: _____

- o Emergency Room: _____

- o Surgery Center: _____

- o Specialty Center: _____

- o Other: _____

Physician: _____

Additional Information:

Via: Phone | Meeting |Other _____

Specialty Physician Name: _____

Office Name: _____

Phone Number: _____

Address: _____

Facility Affiliation:

- o Primary Care Group: _____

- o Hospital: _____

- o Cancer Center: _____

- o Emergency Room: _____

- o Surgery Center: _____

- o Specialty Center: _____

- o Other: _____

SPECIALTY PHYSICIAN: _____

Additional Information:

Page _____ of _____   Via: Phone | Meeting |Other _____

~Healthcare~

Checklist for Hospital Information section:

☐ Hospital Information sheet(s)

A sheet can be filled out for each Hospital. Each sheet should list multiple admissions/Discharges for one facility. It is very important to have all historical visits listed if possible with dates, surgeries, and historical medical records of treatments. Even childhood records if possible.

The more information a physician has, the more of an understanding of the patient he/she can be.

Organizational Notebook #2
"White"

The Gauntlet of Caregiving

Include discharge paperwork in "Healthcare Records"!

HOSPITAL:

Hospital Name:_____

Office Name: _____

Phone Number:_____

Address: _____

- o Emergency Room Date: _____ Discharge Papers Included:___
- o Admission Date: _____ Discharge Date:_____
- o Reason: _____

Hospital Name:_____

Office Name: _____

Phone Number:_____

Address: _____

- o Emergency Room Date: _____ Discharge Papers Included:___
- o Admission Date: _____ Discharge Date:_____
- o Reason: _____

Hospital Name:_____

Office Name: _____

Phone Number:_____

Address: _____

- o Emergency Room Date: _____ Discharge Papers Included:___
- o Admission Date: _____ Discharge Date:_____
- o Reason:_____

Hospital Name:_____

Office Name: _____

Phone Number:_____

Address: _____

- o Emergency Room Date: _____ Discharge Papers Included:___
- o Admission Date: _____ Discharge Date: _____
- o Reason: _____

Hospital Name:_____

Office Name: _____

Phone Number:_____

Address: _____

- o   Emergency Room   Date: _____   Discharge Papers Included:___
- o   Admission   Date: _____   Discharge Date:_____
- o   Reason: _____

Hospital Name:_____

Office Name: _____

Phone Number:_____

Address: _____

- o   Emergency Room   Date: _____   Discharge Papers Included:___
- o   Admission   Date: _____   Discharge Date:_____
- o   Reason: _____

Hospital Name:_____

Office Name: _____

Phone Number:_____

Address: _____

- o   Emergency Room   Date: _____   Discharge Papers Included:___
- o   Admission   Date: _____   Discharge Date:_____
- o   Reason:_____

Hospital Name:_____

Office Name: _____

Phone Number:_____

Address: _____

- o   Emergency Room   Date: _____   Discharge Papers Included:___
- o   Admission   Date: _____   Discharge Date: _____
- o   Reason: _____

~Healthcare~

Checklist for Veterans Health Info. section:

☐ Veterans Administration

This information will provide location and type of treatment received from the VA. Check off the services on the list that matches the location.

Record Physician information in "Physicians" tab, Healthcare Records from VA will be stored in "Healthcare Records" tab, VA Hospital submissions will be recorded in the "Hospitals" tab, VA Rehabilitation services recorded in the "Nursing Home Rehab" tab and VA medical equipment in the "DME Medical Equipment" tab.

Organizational Notebook #2
"White"

The Gauntlet of Caregiving

Veterans Administration: _____

State/County/City: _____

Service Branch(s): _____

Service provided: _____

Contact: _____ **Extension:** _____

Phone Number: _____

Address: _____

○ Veterans' Healthcare Clinic *(Include Physician on Physician Form)*

○ Veterans Hospital *(Include Hospital on Hospital Forms)*

○ Veterans Nursing Home/Rehab *(Include in Nursing Home/Rehab Forms)*

○ Other Specialties *(Include Specialty Physician on Specialty Physician Form)*

○ Prescriptions received from VA? *(Make a note on medication list where refilled)*

○ Aid and Attendance funding

○ Other _____

○ Other _____

○ Other _____

ADDITIONAL INFORMATION:

_____

_____

_____

_____

_____

_____

VETERANS ADMINISTRATION: _____

~Healthcare~

Checklist for Nursing Home/Rehab Info. section:

☐ DME Medical Equipment

A sheet can be filled out for each Nursing Home/Rehab visit. Each sheet should list multiple admissions/Discharges for one facility. It is very important to have all historical visits listed if possible, with dates, reason for admission, and historical medical records of treatments. You will need to ask for discharge records that include Doctor name, medication list and prescriptions for post visit, instructions for followup outside the facility for such professional services as PT, OT, Physicians, etc.

The more information a primary or emergency physician has, the more of an understanding of the patient he/she can be.

Organizational Notebook #2

"White"

Nursing Home/Rehab Name: _____

Office Name: _____

Phone Number:_____

Address: _____

- o Nursing Home Admission Date: _____ Discharge Papers Included:___
- o Rehab Admission   Date: _____ Discharge Date:_____
- o Reason:_____

Nursing Home/Rehab Name: _____

Office Name: _____

Phone Number:_____

Address: _____

- o Nursing Home Admission Date: _____ Discharge Papers Included:___
- o Rehab Admission   Date: _____ Discharge Date:_____
- o Reason:_____

Nursing Home/Rehab Name: _____

Office Name: _____

Phone Number:_____

Address: _____

- o Nursing Home Admission Date: _____ Discharge Papers Included:___
- o Rehab Admission   Date: _____ Discharge Date:_____
- o Reason:_____

Nursing Home/Rehab Name: _____

Office Name: _____

Phone Number:_____

Address: _____

- o Nursing Home Admission Date: _____ Discharge Papers Included:___
- o Rehab Admission   Date: _____ Discharge Date:_____
- o Reason:_____

NURSING HOME/REHAB:

Nursing Home/Rehab Name: _____

Office Name: _____

Phone Number:_____

Address: _____

- o Nursing Home Admission Date: _____   Discharge Papers Included:___
- o Rehab Admission   Date: _____   Discharge Date:_____
- o Reason:_____

Nursing Home/Rehab Name: _____

Office Name: _____

Phone Number:_____

Address: _____

- o Nursing Home Admission Date: _____   Discharge Papers Included:___
- o Rehab Admission   Date: _____   Discharge Date:_____
- o Reason:_____

Nursing Home/Rehab Name: _____

Office Name: _____

Phone Number:_____

Address: _____

- o Nursing Home Admission Date: _____   Discharge Papers Included:___
- o Rehab Admission   Date: _____   Discharge Date:_____
- o Reason:_____

Nursing Home/Rehab Name: _____

Office Name: _____

Phone Number:_____

Address: _____

- o Nursing Home Admission Date: _____   Discharge Papers Included:___
- o Rehab Admission   Date: _____   Discharge Date:_____
- o Reason:_____

NURSING HOME/REHAB:

~Healthcare~

Checklist for DME Medical Equipment section:

☐ *Fill out a sheet for every piece of medical equipment that is provided through every company even though there is a sticker on the equipment, they sometimes fall off or get removed.*

Example: A walker is provided by ABC equipment company, DEF company delivers the equipment and sets up, billing is done through XYZ billing, and SRQ insurance company pays the bill. If the equipment is returned to ABC company and does not notify XYZ billing and SRQ insurance pays for a month when you no longer have the equipment, verification is needed as to when the equipment was surrendered. This form is where to record this information, so you are not personally charged for the equipment. Also if DEF picks up the equipment be sure to ask for a receipt and include this in the "DME Medical Equipment" tab.

Organizational Notebook #2
"White"

DME MEDICAL EQUIPMENT

The Gauntlet of Caregiving

Note: One sheet per piece of DME equipment is recommended.

MEDICAL EQUIPMENT: _____

Medical Equipment Provider: _____

Office name: _____

Phone number: _____

Address: _____

Description of equipment: _____

Rented   Owned   Borrowed

Serviced by:_____

       Service schedule: Weekly   Monthly   On Call

       Last service date: _____

Other information:

_____
_____
_____
_____
_____
_____
_____
_____
_____
_____
_____
_____

Returned date: _____

Where: _____

Signature of receiver: _____
(Recommended)

Additional Information:

Page _____ of _____   Via: Phone | Meeting |Other _____

~Healthcare~

Checklist for Appt. Note Blanks section:

☐ Blank Appointment Note sheets. Keep at least 10 copies ready to go.

Organizational Notebook #2
"White"

The Gauntlet of Caregiving

The Gauntlet of Caregiving – HEALTHCARE - Organizational Notebook 2
These Note Forms move to "Healthcare Records" accompanied by a Summary of Office/Hospital Visit filed in
Chronological Order keeping the most recent information on top for easy access.

1|2|3|4|5|6|7|8|9|10|11|12|13|14|15|16|17|18|19|20|21|22|23|24|25|26|27|28|29|30|31

January | February | March | April | May | June | July | August | September | October | November | December

Monday | Tuesday | Wednesday | Thursday | Friday |Saturday | Sunday

Time: _____ AM | PM

Provider of Service _____ Location _____

Future Appointments: _____ ◯ Same location or ◯ Different location

Location if different: _____

Concerns, Diagnosis, Plan and Notes from this appointment:

_____

_____

_____

_____

_____

_____

_____

_____

_____

_____

_____

_____

_____

_____

_____

_____

_____

_____

Page _____ of _____   Via: Phone | Meeting |Other _____

The Gauntlet of Caregiving – HEALTHCARE - Organizational Notebook 2
These Note Forms move to "Healthcare Records" accompanied by a Summary of Office/Hospital Visit filed in
Chronological Order keeping the most recent information on top for easy access.

Continued

_____

Page _____ of _____   Via: Phone | Meeting | Other _____

~Confidential~
Estate & Legal

Checklist for Attorney & Accountant section:

☐ Complete a form for each Attorney and Accountant. Check off what service(s) are/were provided. Make a note of date of service(s)

Organizational Notebook #3
"Green"

The Gauntlet of Caregiving

Important Essential Information

LOCATOR LIST

This information and its location should be readily available to the person who will be a caregiver if ever needed. Whether a Spouse, Child, Relative or Friend/Guardian, it is imperative that someone has access so that YOU can be taken care of when needed.

If there is a confidence or conflict issue, a third party such as an Attorney or Guardian should be assigned to hold this information.

Identification requirements*	Location
o Driver's License(s) or State Issued ID	o _____
o Social Security Card(s)	o _____
o Birth Certificate	o _____
o Proof of Citizenship or Green card	o _____
o Passport	o _____
o Veteran: DD214	o _____
o Pension Identification Card(s)	o _____
Personal Health Information*	
o Medicare Card(s)	o _____
o Supplemental Health Insurance Cards (Copy front & back)	o _____
o Long Term Health Care Insurance	o _____
o Dental & Vision Insurance	o _____
o Other Health Plans such as VA, Government Employee, or Pension Plans *(Do not copy Government ID's especially Military ID's, it is a violation and illegal)*	o _____
o List of Current Medications, Prescribing Doctor, Use & Dosage (Health History Form)	o _____
o List of Current Doctors or Specialty Care Physician(s) (Health History Form)	o _____
o List of Doctors Recently Scene in Hospital (Health History Form)	o _____
o Health History (Health History Form)	o _____
o Living Will (See Links to State Requirements)	o _____
o Healthcare Directive (See Links to State Requirements)	o _____
o Healthcare Surrogate Designation (See Links to State Requirements)	o _____
o Healthcare Power of Attorney (See Links to State Requirements)	o _____
Personal Assets and Financial Management*	

o Motor Vehicle Registration or Title (Cars, Campers, Motorcycle, Mobile Homes) If financed, Financial Institution information, copy of loan(s) & Payment Information	o _____
o Income Verification from ALL sources including Pension Benefits	o _____
o Checking/Savings, Brokerage accounts, Statements of all for past 3-6 months	o _____
o Income Tax Filing for last 5 yrs.	o _____
o Mortgage Information (Asset Liability Form)	o _____
o Property Tax Bill(s) & Addresses (The property address does not always appear on the bill)	o _____
o Property Insurance Providers (Homeowners, Vehicle, Boat, Camper, Golf Cart, Motorcycle, etc.)	o _____
o Personal Residence and Value (Required for Government programs that are based on assets and income such as Medicaid, County/City in Home Care, & other programs)	o _____
o Technology User Names and Passwords for online accounts.	o _____
o Power of Attorney (Durable and stated powers)	o _____
Legal and Professional*	
o Long-Term Care Insurance Policies	o _____
o Business Papers: Partnership Agreements, Financial Statements, Buy/Sell Agreements	o _____
o Life Insurance and Annuity Policies including current values	o _____
o Funeral Planning Declaration (Include all Details)	o _____
o Trust Agreements or TOD – Transfer on Death Deed for Real Estate	o _____
o Last Will and Testament (Attorney Name or Where is it held)	o _____
o Estate Planning and/or Elder Care Attorney Name and Contact Information	o _____

Attorney/Accountant Name: _____

Office Name: _____

Phone Number: _____

Address: _____

Service Provided:

- ○ Estate Planning – Personal   Date: _____
- ○ Corporate   Date: _____
- ○ Corporate Tax   Date: _____
- ○ Power of Attorney   Date: _____
- ○ Healthcare Directive   Date: _____
- ○ Tax – Personal   Date: _____
- ○ Trust(s)   Date: _____
- ○ Will   Date: _____
- ○ Other: _____   Date: _____
- ○ Other: _____   Date: _____
- ○ Other: _____   Date: _____
- ○ Other: _____   Date: _____

Attorney/Accountant: _____

Additional Information:

_____

_____

_____

_____

_____

_____

_____

Attorney/Accountant Name: _____

Office Name: _____

Phone Number: _____

Address: _____

Service Provided:

- o   Estate Planning – Personal   Date: _____
- o   Corporate   Date: _____
- o   Corporate Tax   Date: _____
- o   Power of Attorney   Date: _____
- o   Healthcare Directive   Date: _____
- o   Tax – Personal   Date: _____
- o   Trust(s)   Date: _____
- o   Will   Date: _____
- o   Other: _____   Date: _____
- o   Other: _____   Date: _____
- o   Other: _____   Date: _____
- o   Other: _____   Date: _____

Attorney/Accountant: _____

Additional Information:

_____

_____

_____

_____

_____

_____

_____

The Gauntlet of Caregiving – Organizational Notebook 3

~Confidential~
Estate & Legal

Checklist for Power of Attorney (POA) section:

☐ This section is designated to store the "Power of Attorney" originals.

☐ There are many different types of these documents :

- *Healthcare POA, copies can be made and placed in the "Power of Attorney" section in Notebook #1 (Purple), the original can be stored here and notebook kept in a secure place.*

- *Financial POA can be kept in this notebook in "Power of Attorney" tab or make a reference to where these documents are kept ie.: Attorney's office referencing "Attorney/Accountant" tab in notebook #3.*

Organizational Notebook #3
"Green"

The Gauntlet of Caregiving

~Confidential~
Estate & Legal

Checklist for Personal Financial section:

- ☐ Banking information
- ☐ Investments with an investment Broker
- ☐ Crypto Currency accounts
- ☐ Any financial institution account information and where to find, who to talk to.
- ☐ Information about how accounts are setup for POA usage.

Organizational Notebook #3
"Green"

The Gauntlet of Caregiving

Banking

Institution Name: _____

Office Name: _____

Phone Number: _____

Address: _____

NOTE: Upon death a POA is no longer valid and bank accounts will be frozen. Accounts should have an alternate option for access. Speak with a Bank Customer Service Professional or an Attorney to use an option such as 'In Trust For,' or additional signor on the account, etc.

Service Provided:

- ○ Checking (Type)_____ Account #: _____
- ○ Checking (Type)_____ Account #: _____
- ○ Checking (Type)_____ Account #: _____
- ○ Checking (Type)_____ Account #: _____
- ○ Checking (Type)_____ Account #: _____
- ○ Checking (Type)_____ Account #: _____
- ○ Savings (Type)_____ Account #: _____
- ○ Savings (Type)_____ Account #: _____
- ○ Savings (Type)_____ Account #: _____
- ○ Savings (Type)_____ Account #: _____
- ○ Other   (Type)_____ Account #: _____
- ○ Other   (Type)_____ Account #: _____

Institution Name: _____

Additional Information:

_____

_____

_____

_____

_____

The Gauntlet of Caregiving – Organizational Notebook 3

Banking

Institution Name: _____

Office Name: _____

Phone Number: _____

Address: _____

NOTE: Upon death a POA is no longer valid and bank accounts will be frozen. Accounts should have an alternate option for access. Speak with a Bank Customer Service Professional or an Attorney to use an option such as 'In Trust For,' or additional signor on the account, etc.

Service Provided:

- Checking (Type)_____   Account #: _____
- Checking (Type)_____   Account #: _____
- Checking (Type)_____   Account #: _____
- Checking (Type)_____   Account #: _____
- Checking (Type)_____   Account #: _____
- Checking (Type)_____   Account #: _____
- Savings (Type)_____   Account #: _____
- Savings (Type)_____   Account #: _____
- Savings (Type)_____   Account #: _____
- Savings (Type)_____   Account #: _____
- Other   (Type)_____   Account #: _____
- Other   (Type)_____   Account #: _____

Institution Name: _____

Additional Information:

_____

_____

_____

_____

_____

The Gauntlet of Caregiving – Organizational Notebook 3

Investment Portfolio

Institution Name: _____

Office Name: _____

Phone Number: _____

Address: _____

Service Provided:

- ○ Investment Portfolio   Date: _____
- ○ Stocks   Date: _____
- ○ Annuity   Date: _____
- ○ Real Property   Date: _____
- ○ Bonds   Date: _____
- ○ Deferred Tax Investments   Date: _____
- ○ Trust(s)   Date: _____
- ○ Other: _____   Date: _____
- ○ Other: _____   Date: _____
- ○ Other: _____   Date: _____
- ○ Other: _____   Date: _____
- ○ Other: _____   Date: _____

Institution Name: _____

Additional Information:

_____

_____

_____

_____

_____

The Gauntlet of Caregiving – Organizational Notebook 3

Investment Portfolio

Institution Name: _____

Office Name: _____

Phone Number: _____

Address: _____

Service Provided:

- ○ Investment Portfolio   Date: _____
- ○ Stocks   Date: _____
- ○ Annuity   Date: _____
- ○ Real Property   Date: _____
- ○ Bonds   Date: _____
- ○ Deferred Tax Investments   Date: _____
- ○ Trust(s)   Date: _____
- ○ Other: _____   Date: _____
- ○ Other: _____   Date: _____
- ○ Other: _____   Date: _____
- ○ Other: _____   Date: _____
- ○ Other: _____   Date: _____

Institution Name: _____

Additional Information:

_____

_____

_____

_____

_____

The Gauntlet of Caregiving – Organizational Notebook 3

ONLINE STOCK/CRYPTCURRENCY TRADING ACCOUNTS

Use one sheet for each trading account.

YOUR NAME: _____   **DATE:** _____

Type of account: Stocks/Basic/Futures   Cryptocurrency/Basic/Contracts Other: _____

Device used:

○ Desktop Computer: Description/Location _____

○ Mobile Phone: Description/Location _____

○ Laptop Computer: Description/Location _____

○ Tablet: Description/Location _____

Software or App(s) used to access and trade assets:

These are a few examples for Cryptocurrencies trading platforms and wallets: crypto.com, Coinbase, Kraken.

These are a few examples for Stock/ETF trading platforms: Robinhood, SoFi, moomoo, J.P.Morgan, TradeStation.

Name of Main Broker Platform/Wallet: _____

Name/User ID: _____

Other ID used (SS#): _____

Password: _____

Name of Secondary Broker Platform/Wallet: _____

Name/User ID: _____

Other ID used (SS#): _____

Password: _____

App for two factor authentication (2fA) if setup using separate app: _____

Name/User ID: _____

Other ID used (SS#): _____

Password: _____

Names of stocks or currencies available to transfer or cashout on this platform/wallet:

Name of Stocks/Cryptocurrencies (Example stocks: Tesla, Apple stocks, Vanguard ETF; Crypto: BTC, ETH, DOGE, BAT, WDL):

_____ _____ _____ _____ _____ _____ _____

_____ _____ _____ _____ _____ _____ _____

_____ _____ _____ _____ _____ _____ _____

_____ _____ _____ _____ _____ _____ _____

_____ _____ _____ _____ _____ _____ _____

_____ _____ _____ _____ _____ _____ _____

_____ _____ _____ _____ _____ _____ _____

_____ _____ _____ _____ _____ _____ _____

Liquid assets stored in wallet/spot: $_____ $_____

Bank account(s) associated with this trading platform:

Name of Bank: _____ Account #: _____

Account name: _____ Password: _____

Other identifying information: _____

Contacts who can help with accessing and securing funds in this account:

Name: _____ Contact phone: _____

Name: _____ Contact phone: _____

Name: _____ Contact phone: _____

Name: _____ Contact phone: _____

Additional Information:

_____

_____

_____

_____

~Confidential~
Estate & Legal

Checklist for Estate Planning section:

- ☐ List of what is included in Estate Planning
- ☐ Copies of Estate Plan or originals or where to locate

Organizational Notebook #3
"Green"

The Gauntlet of Caregiving

Estate Planning Word Definitions

Assets

Generally, anything a person owns, including a home and other real estate, bank accounts, life insurance, investments, furniture, jewelry, art, clothing, and collectibles.

Beneficiary

A person or entity (such as a charity) that receives a beneficial interest in something, such as an estate, trust, account, or insurance policy.

Distribution

A payment in cash or asset(s) to the beneficiary, individual, or entity who is entitled to receive it.

Estate

All assets and debts left by an individual at death.

Fiduciary

A person with a legal obligation (duty) to act primarily for another person's benefit, e.g., a trustee or agent under a power of attorney. "Fiduciary" implies great confidence and trust, and a high degree of good faith.

Funding

The process of transferring (re-titling) assets to a living trust. A living trust will only avoid probate at the trustmaker's death if it is fully funded, meaning it contains all of the decedent's assets.

Incapacitated/Incompetent

Unable to manage one's own affairs, either temporarily or permanently; often involves a lack of mental capacity.

Inheritance

The assets received from someone who has died.

Living probate

The court-supervised process of managing the assets of an incapacitated person. Conservatorship is another term used for this process.

Marital deduction

A deduction on the federal estate tax return, it lets the first spouse to die leave an unlimited amount of assets to the surviving spouse free of estate taxes. However, if no other tax planning is used and the surviving spouse's estate is more than the amount of the federal estate tax exemption in effect at the time of the surviving spouse's death, estate taxes will be due at that time.

Settle an estate

The process of winding down the final affairs (valuation of assets, payment of debts and taxes, distribution of assets to beneficiaries) after someone dies.

Trust

A fiduciary relationship in which one party, known as the trustmaker or settlor, gives another party, known as the trustee, the right to hold property or assets for the benefit of another party, the beneficiary. The trust should be memorialized by a written trust agreement, outlining how the trust assets will be distributed to the beneficiary.

Will

A written document with instructions for disposing of assets after death. A will can only be enforced through a probate court. A will can also contain the nomination of guardian for minor children.

~Confidential~
Estate & Legal

Checklist for Security User ID & Password section:

☐ This is where the user identification and passwords can be kept for all accounts that exist and require secure login.

☐ This list should be updated regularly.

☐ Only inform trusted individuals with where this notebook and information is located. Always speak to an Attorney and if appropriate provide location information to him/her.

SECURITY
UID & PW.

Organizational Notebook #3
"Green"

The Gauntlet of Caregiving

Name/Type of Account	What it is called (Nickname)	Location (File/Device)	Username	Password
Credit Card:				
Credit Card:				
Credit Card:				
Credit Card:				
Credit Card:				
Device: Audio Books				
Device: Computer				
Device: Email 1				
Device: Email 2				
Device: Internet				
Device: Kindle				
Device: Music				
Device: Other				
Device: Phone				
Financial: Assets				
Financial: Assets				
Financial: Checking				
Financial: Mortgage				
Financial: Safety Dep Box				
Healthcare portal: Doctor				
Healthcare portal: Hospital				
Home: House access (alarm)				
Home: Safe access				
Insurance policy: Health				
Insurance policy: Life				
Insurance policy: Other				
Insurance policy: Savings				
Medicare:				
Memberships: Facebook				
Memberships: Modem				

The Gauntlet of Caregiving

Name/Type of Account	What it is called (Nickname)	Location (File/Device)	Username	Password
Memberships: Other				
Memberships: TV Channel				
Memberships: TV Channel				
Memberships: TV Channel				
Memberships: TV Channel				
Memberships: TV Provider				
Memberships: Wifi/Internet				
Social Security:				
Subscriptions:				
Subscriptions:				
Subscriptions:				
Subscriptions: Identity Protection				
Travel Airline CC				
Travel CC				
Travel: AAA, Other				
Travel: AARP, Other				

The Gauntlet of Caregiving

~Confidential~
Estate & Legal

Checklist for Final Arrangements section:

☐ This form will help to facilitate what happens, who to contact, final arrangement information and loving messages from the person who has passed.

A very emotional but important section to complete!

Organizational Notebook #3
"Green"

The Gauntlet of Caregiving

--------------------*Final Arrangements*--------------------
Know I love you and
thank you for
taking care of things for me.

It is important that this information has been kept up to date. If a policy is cashed out or changed it should be X out and updated information should be added. If the policy is for health insurance updates changes should also be made in the "Personal Health Information" section of the "Organizational Notebook 2." This information should also match the Username and Password sheet.

Legal Name: First _____ Middle _____ Last _____

Married Name: First _____ Middle _____ Last _____

Married Name: First _____ Middle _____ Last _____

Married Name: First _____ Middle _____ Last _____

Alias: (PhD, MD, etc.) _____

Birth Name: First _____ Middle _____ Last _____

Date of Birth: _____ USA Citizen: Y N   Military Veteran: Y N Branch: _____

Birth State: _____ Country: _____ Province _____

SS#: _____ Green card carrier: Y N ID number: _____

Benefits from another Country? Y N ID number: _____ _____

Date of Death: _____ City/County/State: _____

Last Home Address: _____City/State/Zip: _____

Primary Address: Y N (If no, provide additional information)

Primary Home Address: _____ City/State/Zip: _____

Other (Description Name of Business/Contact Name/etc.) _____

Address: _____ City/State/Zip: _____

What to do when I am gone.

Who to Contact, Names are listed on following pages:

1. Contact a family member or friend to help, please.
2. Contact the Funeral Home and/or Organization of Donorship.
3. Contact other family members and friends to let them know.
4. Notify employer or volunteer group(s) who may be expecting me.
5. Contact the Attorney to consult regarding obligations and the will.

What needs to be done:

1. Setup arrangements, according to my wishes, with the funeral home.
2. Order at least 10 original copies of the death certificate from funeral home.
3. Contact Social Security to stop benefits.*
4. Contact Life and Health Insurance Companies to inform.*
5. Contact Pension Funds, Annuities, Asset Managers, Stockbrokers*
6. Contact Financial institutions (Debt: Bank, Mortgage Company, Credit Card Companies)*
7. Place a notification in the newspaper, affiliation newsletters and online.

*Income: Some income benefits may cease or require refund depending on the date of payment vs the date of death. Be prepared to refund if the payor requires it. Insurance: if a premium for insurance is not paid, make sure to keep paying until they indicate in writing it is no longer necessary. Otherwise it could affect benefits. Financials: All asset managers need to be immediately notified so that no assets can be fraudulently disbursed. Debt Management: Notify these institutions who will be paying. Executor of Will: Consult the Attorney of record if a Will is in place. If the Attorney is named as Executor of the Will, he/she will instruct how to proceed. If someone else is named Executor of the Will it is important to include instructions from a reputable source what steps need to be taken to settle the estate. Here are a few, but not all questions, to ask and have answered. NOTE: this is not financial or legal advice.

- How do I sell someone else's car or other titled possessions after the power of attorney is no longer valid?
- How do I settle debt after the power of attorney is no longer valid and if funds are frozen at the bank.
- Do I need to set up a separate account for the Estate?
- What do I do if there is no will or executor designated, and the power of attorney is no longer valid?

Final Arrangements:

Funeral Home: _____ Address: _____

Phone: _____Ext. _____ Contact Name: _____

Policy/Contract Location: _____

Other (Newspaper, Online Dignity/Ancestry/Legacy): _____

Address: _____ City/State/Zip: _____

Phone: _____Ext. _____ Contact Name: _____

Policy/Contract/Designation Location: _____

Other (Crematorium, Neptune Society, Donor): _____

Address: _____ City/State/Zip: _____

Phone: _____Ext. _____ Contact Name: _____

Policy/Contract/Designation Location: _____

Other (Crematorium, Neptune Society, Donor): _____

Address: _____ City/State/Zip: _____

Phone: _____Ext. _____ Contact Name: _____

Policy/Contract/Designation Location: _____

Other (Crematorium, Neptune Society, Donor): _____

Address: _____ City/State/Zip: _____

Phone: _____Ext. _____ Contact Name: _____

Policy/Contract/Designation Location: _____

Family & Friends

Name: _____ Address: _____

Phone: _____ Relation: _____ Email: _____

Name: _____ Address: _____

Phone: _____ Relation: _____ Email: _____

Name: _____ Address: _____

Phone: _____ Relation: _____ Email: _____

Name: _____ Address: _____

Phone: _____ Relation: _____ Email: _____

Name: _____ Address: _____

Phone: _____ Relation: _____ Email: _____

Business/Professional Affiliations:

Name: _____ Address: _____

Phone: _____ Relation: _____ Email: _____

Name: _____ Address: _____

Phone: _____ Relation: _____ Email: _____

Name: _____ Address: _____

Phone: _____ Relation: _____ Email: _____

Name: _____ Address: _____

Phone: _____ Relation: _____ Email: _____

If no other arrangements have been made, please use this information.

My favorite Music/Songs: _____

Favorite Movies: _____

Favorite Photograph(s) Location: _____

Religion/Prayer(s) Name or Location:_____

Additional Information:

_____

_____

_____

_____

_____

Insurance & Benefit Policies *in Alphabetical Order*

Accidental Death Insurance:

Insurance Provider: _____ Policy Number: _____

Additional: _____ Policy Number: _____

Insurance Provider: _____ Policy Number: _____

Additional: _____ Policy Number: _____

Auto Insurance:

- Insurance Provider: _____ Policy Number: _____
  Location: _____

- Insurance Provider: _____ Policy Number: _____
  Location: _____

- Insurance Provider: _____ Policy Number: _____
  Location: _____

Health Insurance: (Medicare, Medicaid, Private, Employer) If blank, refer to Locator List.

- Insurance Provider: _____ Policy Number: _____
  Location of Policy: _____
  Coverage In Use: _____

- Insurance Provider: _____ Policy Number: _____
  Location of Policy: _____
  Coverage In Use: _____

- Insurance Provider: _____ Policy Number: _____
  Location of Policy: _____
  Coverage In Use: _____

- Insurance Provider: _____ Policy Number: _____
  Location of Policy: _____
  Coverage In Use: _____

Long Term Care Insurance:

- Insurance Provider: _____ Policy Number: _____
  Location of Policy: _____
  Coverage In Use: _____

Life Insurance:

- Insurance Provider (Employer/Pension/etc): _____
  Insurance Company: _____ Policy Number: _____
  Type: _____ Use: _____
  Location of Policy: _____
- Insurance Provider (Employer/Pension/etc): _____
  Insurance Company: _____ Policy Number: _____
  Type: _____ Use: _____
  Location of Policy: _____

Property & Business Insurances:

- Property Address/City/State: _____
  Insurance Provider: _____ Policy Number: _____
  Type: _____ Use: _____
  Location of Policy: _____

- Property Address/City/State: _____
  Insurance Provider: _____ Policy Number: _____
  Type: _____ Use: _____
  Location of Policy: _____

- Property Address/City/State: _____
  Insurance Provider: _____ Policy Number: _____
  Type: _____ Use: _____
  Location of Policy: _____

- Property Address/City/State: _____
  Insurance Provider: _____ Policy Number: _____
  Type: _____ Use: _____
  Location of Policy: _____

Additional Information such as previous or alternative address history, location of items not previously or otherwise disclosed. Date these items if necessary for legal purposes.

Additional Information continued:

~Confidential~
Estate & Legal

Checklist for Last Will & Testament section:

☐ A copy, the original or reference to where this document is located. Use 'Locator List of Important Information' if documents are not kept here.

Organizational Notebook #3
"Green"

The Gauntlet of Caregiving

~Confidential~
Estate & Legal

Checklist for Miscellaneous Documents section:

☐ This section is for "Miscellaneous Original" documents that may not match any other category in Notebook #3.

☐ Examples would be:

- DD2-14 Military Service Document

- Official Retirement Benefit Qualification Documentation

- Certification of Citizenship

- Birth Certificate

- Marriage Certificate

- Divorce Documentation

- Pre-paid Burial Contract/Receipts

  (Make a note on "Final Arrangements" form)

Use 'Locator List of Important Information' if documents are not kept here.

Organizational Notebook #3
"Green"

MISC. ORIGINAL DOCUMENTS

The Gauntlet of Caregiving